DICKY GALORE

SEX-*capades*
By The Decades
The Twenties

EPIC PRESS

Published by:
Epic Press
PO Box 30108
Walnut Creek, CA 94598
First *Epic Press* Edition published 2–007

Fondly dedicated
with mightily throbbing
love and affection
to
every sweet *Pussy Galore*
everywhere(or to all the
sweet *Pussy Galores*)I've
loved before!

CONTENTS

PROLOGUE:
(The Teaser)
LOVE LOST,
VIRGINITY GIVEN

"I ruined my chance for happiness with you. I wonder if I will ever be that happy again."—**Regina, 11 March 1974**

Long Beach, Mississippi 3 February 1974

One day before the so-called *Symbionese Liberation Army* kidnapped from Berkeley, California newspaper heiress Patricia Hearst, I hurtled headlong into the jaws of death, and like a bat out of hell, winged my way right out again scot-free! Such is the unbelievably good fortune of any aspiring superspy–like hero all of 20, barreling along the Mississippi Gulf Coast in stormy weather at breakneck speed like some daring, daredevil stunt driver!

That cloudy and gusty stretch of Interstate Highway 10 was being drenched in blustering, torrential rain. My sweaty palms lightly gripped the steering wheel of my fresh-ly painted, blue–green, four–door 1967 *Ford Mercury Comet* as it sped west–bound down the right–hand lane of the rain–soaked road. I squinted, peering intently through the rain–spattered windshield being cleared only fleetingly by squeaky wipers. Storm–churned breakers surging all along the billowing seashore whisked by. My car was racing over treacherous, slippery ground. All four of its treadless tires were bald as billiard balls. And I was driving recklessly—fast and furious—like some rash and silly lovesick young fool all excited to visit my recently *old* high school sweetheart.

Unexpectedly my car started skimming across the slick sheet of rainwater flooding the road—its wheels locked solid! It was hydroplaning! My foot pumped the brake pedal, first slightly and then frantically without any effect! Slamming the pedal flat to the floorboard was futile! My brakes were completely gone! And my car was careening across that rain–soused surface completely out of control!

At one fell swoop I was struck dumb with full force by

11

that terrifying, paralyzing sensation of utter helplessness. Doubtless my jaw dropped, my eyes popped and my breathing stopped as both my hands tightly clenched the steering wheel and both my feet pressed forcefully against the floorboard, bracing for collision. Tenaciously I held on tight for dear life!

Suddenly my screeching car swerved and swung uncontrollably from side to side—fish–tailing!—spinning round and round like a twirling top tail–end first! Sudsy surf, sandy beach and falling rain whirled all around me with a tortuously dizzying but dreamy frenzy! At that instant I truly thought I was dead! And then I was staring—severely startled—glaringly *sky*ward! My car was abruptly *airborne*, capsizing upside down in cloud–clapped space! Rolling in mid–air, it overturned completely before crashing down hard and heavily onto its battered chassis!

When the sand settled, my car had ground to a fast but tilted halt—its front end plunged deeply into a sandy bank, its rear end bulging slantwise from the right shoulder of the road. It was deathly quiet inside that car compartment. Softly hissing steam fumed outside from the crumpled up hood, radiator and grille half–buried in the sand.

Finally I let out all my bated breath with one long–drawn–out softly whistling hiss of my own. In spite of wearing no over–sanctified seat belt—my car wasn't even equipped with one—I hadn't budged an inch from my rooted seat. I was still very much alive and breathing if not kicking. To my overwhelming relief I felt no pain and was wholly unharmed. I had expected but miraculously escaped dying a violent death in a catastrophic car crash. Even more miraculous had been colliding with no other solid fixed object like a telephone pole or another motor vehicle. I'd just turned a complete somersault in pouring rain with my car, landing upright square on its wheels again, and was about to climb out of the wreck completely unscathed!

Strangely the car motor was still running. Calmly I turned off the ignition to stop the quietly idling engine—afraid gasoline might ignite a fire or explosion. Wrenching the handle I found the driver's door jammed shut and was unable to budge it open. So I anxiously clambered over the front seat and onto the back to get out through the right rear door.

Just as I was getting to my feet outside another car was slowing down from behind and pulling up on the shoulder of the road nearby. A kindly, elderly black couple got out of their carefully parked car and reluctantly came up to me with shared expressions of amazement exchanged between them.

"We thought you were dead!" they chimed in unison with bewildered disbelief.

I just stood aghast at my wreck of an automobile, gesturing to it with outstretched hands.

"Look at my car!" I exclaimed.

"Look at *you!*" they exclaimed in turn. "You're lucky to be alive!"

"Well," I said with all the cool and smiling nonchalance I could muster, "could you perhaps give me a lift to the nearest garage to get a tow?"

§

They would indeed drive me back and drop me off with caring and concerned well wishes at a **B&G Standard Oil** service station—owned by Bob Dunn and Gene Reese—situated along the eastward beachfront; and as luck would have it also happened to be a 24–hour towing service agent for the *American Automotive Association(**AAA**)*auto club! Bob's surname was indeed seemly(if not seamy)since he would literally *DUN* me for a service shakedown mounting up to $150.10, including parts and labor, for four new *Goodyear* tires as well as miscellaneous parts(clamps, hose, valve stem, wheel)for the battered radiator which sustained the most disabling damage; I paid their $30 tow charge on the spot. They would tip themselves with the self–confiscated gratuity of my car's *Allied* model 23–channel citizen's band radio(and antenna no less!)and then vociferously blame *me* for leaving it to get un–*bolted* and stolen from the protective custody of their service station parking lot(which Mr *DUN*&Co claimed belonged to the adjacent property of a *National Food Store*)in my absence awaiting my car's makeshift repair.

Nowadays the moniker for Long Beach, Mississippi is known as the so–called "Friendly City." Back then I would've been more inclined to christen it the *THIEVERY* City! That *Radio Shack* CB had cost me a grand total of $135.30. Ironically I had sold for scrap my very first car—a used 1956 blue *Ford* bomb—to raise the cash required to pay for the radio, which I purchased from the retail electronics chain Thursday the 24th of June 1971 so I could participate in Pensacola, Florida's "Blue Angels Radio Assistance Club Inc," which was part of the "Radio Emergency Associated Citizens Teams"(*REACT*), a voluntary radio emergency civic club. But Mr *DUN*&Co could care less about the civic-mindedness of a kid whose CB radio they'd rip off to pad even further their shakedown repair profits—as if *Standard Oil Company* hadn't already gouged and fleeced enough un-suspecting victims over the years through its various, nefari-ous coercive monopoly–instigated anti–trust activities!

Over the next couple months following the theft I'd go through the rigmarole of wasted motions appealing to the company to replace the "alleged loss" of my swiped ra-dio through an insurance liability claim—responsibility for which Mr *DUN*&Company craftily evaded by deliberately parking my repaired automobile on that supermarket lot ad-jacent to their leased service station!

At the time of that car somersault stunt my *Ford Mercury Comet*'s odometer recorded its mileage at 40,441—if we're to trust Mr *DUN*&Co's predatory billing invoice. I had purchased that car used in June 1972 from a major(and supposedly reputable)automobile dealership at 3401 Navy Boulevard in Pensacola, Florida—the so-called "Men of Integrity" at the *Vince Whibbs Pontiac Co*—whose retail installment contract had been so kindly co-signed by my dearly beloved band director at *Pensacola Catholic High School*(**CHS**): **Mr Billy K Reed**—also known to our band most fondly and endearingly as simply "BK" or "Buddha" in honor of his rather portly and stout tummy upon which he'd habitually rest his baton-brandishing arm!

That summer as well Mr Reed had most charitably taken me into his home at 306 Washington Street in Gulf Breeze(a suburb situated to the north across Pensacola Bay on the Fairpoint Peninsula in Santa Rosa County)to live following graduation since I'd left an extremely broken and dysfunctional "home" situation at just 17 at the start of my high school senior year. We'd formed an exceptionally close father–and–son–like bond over the previous four years while I'd practiced fanatically to progress and advance through the brass ranks—under his sage and generous musical tutelage—from last chair–third section to first chair–first section lead trumpet of our high school band! That entire transaction was something of a family affair since the dealership owner's daughter, Kathleen Whibbs, was even a member of my very high school senior class!

Those were also the melodic days of Burt Bacharach–and–Hal David lyrics when that other not–so–full–of–integrity–either local car dealer personality, Ted Ciano of *Ted Ciano Ford*, appeared spieling on local television to the touching contralto *Carpenters'* tune, *They Long To Be Close To You*, his delightfully ugly face enshrouded in blurred and dreamy cloud effects!

We'd both stood aghast at the contract signing when my shyster used car salesman(RB "Eddie" Edmunds)ushered

us into the somber office of the not–so–big man himself—
Vince Whibbs Sr—to be confronted and put on the spot by
being interrogated in front of a witness(son and University
of Florida–indoctrinated attorney, Vince Whibbs Jr)about
whether we entertained any misgivings or reservations con-
cerning the purchase.

And with considerable cause: that used hunk–'o–junk
epitomized the term *"LEMON"* from the word git–go!
And by the time of my daring car somersault stunt I'd already mis–spent considerably more than the 18 monthly
contract installment payments of $47.32 at 414 North
Pace Boulevard to Pensacola's *Midland–Guardian*(finance)
Corporation on profuse and redundant auto repairs! Just recently the car had received a re–spray at *Ace Body Shop* at
3601 Mobile Highway. What was worse, my *State Farm
Mutual Automobile Insurance Company*(with Pensacola agent,
Roger Q Bennett)policy's collision coverage had just recently
lapsed and my car's unsightly(and costly)front–end damage
would go permanently *un*repaired!

So for that aspiring superspy youth that fateful car crash
and subsequent radio rip–off was just another in a long line
of reality doses afflicting me with some conspicuously severe
growing pains!

But what exclusively male character flaw had drawn me
to that particular Gulf Coast highway juncture at that particular point in time in the first place? One that would severely bedevil and vex me throughout the major part of my
aspiring superspy sexploits career: constantly suffering the
dire consequences of letting my remarkably powerful and
virile(and often uncontrollable)male *TOOL*, rather than
my male *brain*, do the majority of my *thinking* for me where
women were concerned!

§

SEXCAPADES

My senior year at *Pensacola Catholic High School* was a rather turbulent if not tumultuous time for me. At just 17 I'd permanently left my abusive and violent dysfunctional "home"—a simple cinderblock house at 605 Edison Drive in the rather grandiose–and–stately–sounding *"Mayfair Estates"*—a working–class neighborhood on the west side of the rather backwater town of Pensacola situated in the Florida panhandle some 50 miles east of Mobile, Alabama. It's no wonder residents regularly referred to Pensacola as being part of the "Redneck Riviera" bible–belt's "Alabama Annex!" Leaving that evil hell–hole finally and for good was long time in coming but, for me, not a moment too soon!

Meddling and supposedly sage and wiser "adults" would admonish me to remain at "home" with my so–called "parents," but as I would admonish them in turn, they hadn't had to live there, I had; and if they wanted to live there and suffer the pain I had then they were more than welcome to it! As for me, I was finally out of there once and for all and never once regretted it for even a single *nanosecond*—then or since! Living there had been for years an unadulterated hell–on–earth for a sensitive and "soft–hearted"(the words of my own bastard step–father)kid such as myself; and I was finally—at long last!—well out of it!

I'd tried leaving the year before as a kid of 16 but that bastard step–father had dragged me back and socked me down to the floor with his ham–handed fist at the carport door to that hellish house in front of my coldly indifferent bitch of a mother, who sat nearby watching approvingly, rocking gently in her creaking black recliner chair, jeering haughtily and curtly remarking, *"Good!"* Force—violent brute force—was all that bastard(whom upon their sole meeting even my soft–spoken high school band director had most diplomatically described as "rough–shod") knew! Well, that bastard and bitch have both been *dead* now for a long while, and *that's "good!"* too, but all so much brackish water under the proverbial bridge by this time!

This time though I was determined and hell–bent on escaping that evil hell–hole come hell or high water; I would and I did! This time, at that definitive moment on the eve of my high school senior year, I was grimly resolved and wouldn't be coerced, forced, or overbearingly intimidated by that bastard step–father any longer to do anything against my free will—ever again! This time I'd unflinchingly planned my escape well. This time I'd arranged for a safe(and secret) place to stay and another friend from my high school band to pick up me and my meager belongings in his mustard yellow *Chevrolet Corvair* to take me there—only this time under the token and not–so–protective but sufficiently serviceable supervision of an Escambia County deputy sheriff! And for once I'd caught that bastard quite off guard and profoundly and rejoicefully reveled in watching a rather stumped if not stupid and dumbstruck expression flush his whole reddened bastard face!

Many kind and generous friends and neighbors who'd long since known me from childhood had lent me their extremely charitable aid and comfort throughout this critical trial in my life. To them I would forever owe an incalculable debt of outright gratitude that would be unrepayable but perpetually and passionately appreciated! And one of my rather dispassionately impassioned supporters during this grievous ordeal was my recently *old* high school sweetheart to whom I was then rushing recklessly into near deadly disaster to see!

Regina was a rather petite little girl who, standing alongside me at six–foot–two, came up roughly to my shoulder–height. Like me she was of certain Italian extraction though quite unlike me, and for that matter my father, she wasn't possessed of darkly Italian features; my own paternal grandmother, Malvina, had in fact emigrated to Boston, Massachusetts straight from Naples, Italy, making me second generation Italian.

SEXCAPADES

Regina was possessed of a good–natured personality and a gentle, sweet oval face, having soft, shoulder–length, fair brown hair, high cheekbones, a rather goodly nose, discerning eyes set beneath rather bushy brows and supple lips that were full though not of the luscious variety and degree I would come in the fullness of time to revere and prefer. By no means beautiful or even comely in the classical sense she was nevertheless pretty if in a rather plain, homely and even graceful way. She looked her cutest when she smiled, deeply dimpling her soft cheeks and exposing her pair of equally crooked upper canine teeth. In her eyes especially she looked something like an unadorned version of actress Brooke Shields. And during my high school senior year I would rather reluctantly but surely come to fall deeply and passionately in love with her, soundly smitten with all the intensely emotional infatuation of adolescent youth.

By her own account I'd first taken notice of Regina at the end of July 1971 when I visited on Garden Street her family's *Premier* bakery business, for which she worked their customer service counter, while I labored under duress nearby at my bastard step–father's independent moving–and–storage company warehouse on Tarragona Street, *Pensacola Movers*. On brief breaks from my involuntary summer servitude I would frequently relish visiting the bakery to heartily partake of their scrumptious cinnamon rolls thickly incrusted with rich creamy white icing.

Having three siblings, one a younger brother, Regina was the youngest of three sisters—one of whom was named Toni Marie, a member of my own high school senior class whom I'd casually dated a couple of times, and for whom I'd actually acted as campaign manager for her failed one–time bid for high school class president. Sometime during that fateful summer though it was Regina who'd somehow, inexplicably, become enamored of me enough to rather forcibly impose upon me both her attentions and affections—clinging to me tenaciously to utter distraction, overcoming my frequently irritable resistance!—until I'd succumbed and finally felt, in turn, rather compelled to become endeared to her; she'd worn me down with her interminably *LONG* talks!

By the time I'd first fled my dysfunctional family "home," Regina had already become my most secret confederate and confidant, picking me up early on weekday mornings at the residence of a fellow disabled, wheelchair–bound *REACT* radio club dispatcher with whom I was temporarily lodging and nursing; and then driving us both to our high school in her sporty *Plymouth Duster.*

By the summer of 1973, when at 19 I'd become wholly self–sufficient and on my own, I'd live in the meantime on the generous largesse of *four* different families, paying them rather token recompense for my support from my minimum wages earned working at various odd jobs. And from a discreet distance, Regina would see me through it all until a lot later on over roughly the next three years, when she'd manage to deliberately distance herself *from* me enough to provoke me ultimately to undertake my habitual, lifelong, sexually–addicted, aspiring superspy sexploits! And even though we were both relatively virtuous and virginal, and never actually made love with one another, Regina would indeed come to symbolically personify my sexual springboard!

Up to a point ours was the classical star–crossed, rich girl–poor boy, Romeo–and–Juliet–style romance: we both passionately declared and proclaimed our endlessly eternal and undying love for one another(and one another *only*). We dearly, deeply and truly loved one another(and one another *only*)very, *very* much, always and forever—more than *any*thing and *any*one else in the whole wide world—and would do *any*thing and *every*thing to be and stay together always and forever, for all time, all the time, never ever to part or lose one another! We would always and forever love, want and need one another(and one another *only*)—and belong to-

20

tally and completely to one another(and one another *only*)—and *nothing* would ever, *ever* alter, destroy or otherwise do away with that love! We'd ultimately and couldn't wait to marry one another—and could never, *ever* live without one another—and our everlasting and neverending love would endure always and forever and would never, *ever* fade away or die! And no one else could ever, ever possibly replace the other—*ever!*

MAYBE!!PROBABLY!!!

Or so—with such a restrictive provision—would Regina typically qualify her extremely conditional professions of unconditional love. It's no wonder then that Regina would grow up in later adult life to become a contracts attorney! *To dream the impossible dream* was a most apt epithet where our relationship was concerned.

In reality Regina was quite the spoilt little brat, admittedly accustomed to ever so many creature comforts and was, indeed, her daddy's special and over–privileged little baby girl. What with her father's bakery business and her mother's thriving social catering business, Regina's hardworking parents were pretty prosperous and well–to–do, living in a spacious split–level house at 2501 North Whaley Avenue in a fairly affluent suburb near *Bayou Texar*, a favored boating basin opening up to Pensacola Bay on the wealthier *East Hill* side of town. They even owned a modest, driveway–docked cabin cruiser craft in which they boated on the bay, taking regular weekend cruises which Regina constantly complained were excursions of sheer arduous drudgery.

On occasion Regina alluded rather mysteriously to certain unspoken and unexplained things about her family that I ought to know about and become aware of were I ever to seriously consider becoming a member of her family! Her ominous intimations smacked of something sinister–like and Mafia–affiliated(well, her father did collaborate with the fraternal Catholic *Knights of Columbus*, posturing in costume regularly in the town's *Mardis Gras* and *Fiesta of Five Flags* festival parades if that counts!). This family most definitely fancied themselves to be members of the elite upper crust of society. Had they lived in feudal times they doubtless would've been part of the landed gentry and titled aristocracy.

They were doubtless adroit at networking in clubby social circles. Why even Regina, who at high school always acted so irritatingly official, baby–sat for the lay high school principal's brats and was even chauffeured by our high school student counselor to *Loyola University* in New Orleans for her music scholarship piano audition. She'd even boast of supposedly attracting the amorous attentions of both a slimy young secular trigonometry teacher(who derided organized religion though parochial school paid his teaching salary)as well as an even slimier young priest who celebrated Masses with a roving microphone like a pontifical Phil Donahue, the preachy TV talk–show host; and who later on was actually defrocked for running off with a young female parishioner!

After becoming more acquainted and familiar with Regina's family I would even volunteer to work for hours along with her—free and for nothing, mind you, except for the dubious privilege of Regina's company in a safe setting acceptable to her parents—on her mother's various social catering functions, typically banquets and wedding receptions carried on at the town's elegant *Garden Center*, simply to be near her.

Naturally Regina's parents never minded exploiting my unpaid employee labor at any of those fatiguing functions—despite their rather spurious claim that I supposedly never paid *them* proper "respect." What they did vociferously object and take strong exception to was my increasingly romantic relationship with their sweet, innocent little daughter—adamantly opposing and protesting against it(and us) from the start!

That relationship pretty much peaked toward the end of my high school senior year while Regina, who was still a junior, amorously accompanied me to my senior prom, permitting me to cop at least one feel of her bosom afterwards in our car parked at her neighborhood's serene *Bayview Park*—before that is getting busted by some voyeuristic, flashlight–wielding cop keeping the city safe for celibacy!

In that spring of 1972 we spent at least three rather rapturous days mostly alone together on my high school senior band trip to the Gainesville, Florida environs with Regina, a privately–tutored pianist, showing up late to accompany me playing my trumpet for state solo competition at which I earned an Excellent(or "High" II)performance rating. After I graduated from high school as a *National Honor Society* student and commenced attending the local *Pensacola Junior College(PJC)*we were prohibited from dating by Regina's parents, who forbade us from seeing or even telephoning each other. Following my graduation then we were relegated to sneaking: exchanging mostly argumentative love letters through either the post or couriers who also happened to be two of Regina's supposedly best friends, Debra and Tina. To her great credit though Regina would forgo going to her own high school senior prom—more in defiance to her parents than out of any misplaced loyalty to me.

As fate would have it during that summer of 1973, following Regina's own high school senior graduation, I would manage at 19 to embark entirely on my own and actually rent an exceptionally cramped garage space room located literally a single block away from Regina's house at 2211 North Whaley Avenue where she lived with her parents and siblings. Throughout all the time I'd resided alone in that cloistered little room—atop a residential driveway in sight of the beautiful bayou across the avenue—Regina would never ever, except once(very briefly), deign to appear or otherwise arrive at my doorstep to visit or spend some private and solitary time with me. That was much too unlady–like a suggestion to even entertain. And I remained there alone until traveling to Washington DC to attend winter semester at the *George Washington University(GWU)*in January 1975!

In the meantime Regina prepared to relocate herself to New Orleans at the Jesuit *Loyola University* where she was awarded a scholarship and to which I myself considered applying—again simply to be near her. When it came to being and staying together in everlasting love for all eternity Regina talked the talk but seldom walked the walk! By the time she enrolled at university in the fall of 1973 she quickly became the big shot college co–ed on campus—all giddy with the neophyte experience of drunken dormitory keg parties and pseudo–intellectual lecture hall histrionics—and got way too big for her academic britches to pay that much attention to me—until her winter semester of 1974 when scholastic things, whether curricular or extracurricular, somehow went inexplicably wrong and she came griping and whining in letters, pleading with me to love and visit her again.

As a prime example, she pestered me no end all throughout her own high school senior year to possess and sport my own high school senior class ring; but by her first semester at university she voiced guilt–ridden doubts about both her self–professed love for me and whether she could remain faithful to what that ring would represent. She even rejected as unrealistic the notion of *weekly* long–distance telephone calls between us while she was away at university. Throughout her first semester there she took up with some character named Fred whom she boasted about cavorting with until he transferred to another school by the winter.

The bottom–line verdict regarding our relationship reduced to the supreme superficiality: *money!* Her parents disapproved of me because I was poor and Regina wouldn't defy her stern and perennially scowling parents in mortal fear of being cut off from their controlling purse strings. So much for fighting for what you want as she'd so spuriously preached.

Regina became quite the expert head–game player and would lamely attempt to string me along—with profuse but false promises of togetherness—to no avail until nearly spring of 1974. By then, and well *before* then, I'd already gotten plenty tired and fed up with being played for a fool in her immature emotional games. And by the time I'd overturned my car on that rainy and slippery Mississippi road in early February 1974, hurrying headlong to cross that 200–mile stretch of Gulf Coast highway between Pensacola and New Orleans to visit Regina one last time at *Loyola University*, unbeknownst to her I'd already taken quite a strong defiant stand(*lying down!*)of my own against her mealy–mouthed game–playing: roughly some *six months* earlier at the end of August 1973 I'd already fully de–virginized myself by sleeping with an incredibly voluptuous young black woman of 32 named Helen!

ONE:

LIVE

AND

LET

LIE

*"I must say you have crossed my mind so many, many times, and sometimes I have wished for your company. I must say that you meant something special to me..."—**Helen, 5 February 1975***

Live and Let Die(1973), starring the suave and sophisticated English actor Sir Roger Moore in his debut outing as not–so–secret British agent James Bond 007, and featuring its exciting title theme song performed by Paul McCartney's *Wings*, was for me anyway the runaway blockbuster movie—released in June—of summer 1973!

Now I love and revere the impeccably handsome, elegant, polished and smooth Sir Roger Moore, but I'm afraid he never did and never could believably embody the most celebrated literary and cinematic superspy ever created, any more than James Bond's truest, purest and most definitive cinematic incarnation, Sir Sean Connery, could conceivably and convincingly portray Simon Templar(the "Saint") whom Sir Roger Moore personified so perfectly on British series television from 1962 to 1969! Nevertheless, Sir Roger Moore's debut performance in that remarkably frisky all–action film was itself rousingly energetic, hip, cool, witty and perfectly *FUN!*

Bosomy Madeline Smith(as Miss Caruso), who mightily upped the ante for Bond girls eye candy when she got her zipper peeled by Bond's magnetic watch—"sheer magnetism, darling!"—was a sumptuous feast for the eyes in *Hammer Horror's Taste the Blood of Dracula(1970)*as Dolly, *The Vampire Lovers(1970)*as Emma Morton, *Frankenstein and the Monster From Hell(1974)*as Sarah, as well as in Vincent Price's dreadfully disappointing *Theater of Blood(1973)*as Rosemary. Sir Roger recommended Madeline to be cast as Miss Caruso after her impressive appearance as Carla in his British television series, *The Persuaders!(1971)*.

Robert Dix(Hamilton), son of Richard Dix, is the veteran of several notable low–budget cult horror flicks, playing amongst them Detective Dillon in *Frankenstein's Daughter(1958)*, Johnny in *Blood of Dracula's Castle(1969)*and Dr Manning in *Horror of the Blood Monsters(1970)*.

Those early 1970s epitomized(and urbanized)the so-called "Blaxploitation" era, featuring principally black talent with Afro hairstyles set to funk and soul music, which that particular Bond film exploited, so to speak, to the utmost. This was the incredibly entertaining prime time period for the incomparable likes of actors Richard Roundtree as *Shaft(1971)*, Ron O'Neal as *Superfly(1972)*and the unsurpassed and supremely sublime actress, Pam Grier, as *Coffy(1973)*and *Foxy Brown(1974)!* Black was beautiful and, so far as I was concerned, full and fleshy black feminine busts were beautiful—most especially then in that era of the now sorely missed feminine halter top! And none were more fully womanly than Pam Grier!

Though these fun flicks never seemed to take themselves or their cartoonishly violent and sexy escapades too very seriously, latter–day critics still harpingly whine ad nauseam about all the "racist stereotypes" they supposedly engendered. Well, quite secure in the confidence that I personally wasn't possessed of any of the so–called "racist" attitudes of the crooked and corrupt white characters typically depicted, I was one white "cracker–honky" dude who was never, ever once offended by the perfect fun to be had enjoying those films and all their remarkably color*ful* characters! To me there are, were and never, ever shall be in existence any so–called "people of color." In "Blaxploitation" flicks both black and white people were color*ful* enough to combine, commingle and cross equally the entire color spectrum. And commingle they did! "Rainbow coalition" indeed!

Besides, those very same Johnny–come–lately critics deliberately warp such concepts as "racist stereotypes," whose real meaning they're totally ignorant of, misinterpreting and misrepresenting them for self–serving politically correct purposes. So they cunningly confuse "stereotypes" with the frequently accurate *generalizations* upon which they might be based, just as they cunningly confuse "racism" with simple *prejudice*, contriving to make them falsely signify one or the other.

A major case–in–point was all their harping whining about the supposedly "stereotypical" and "racist" character of excruciatingly southern Sheriff JW Pepper as expertly portrayed by the exceptionally talented New York character actor, Clifton James. Well, I've got some news for ya'll boys: I've lived in the deep bible–belt south for roughly two decades and can personally attest from many a personal encounter with southern cops that Clifton's comical characterization— and southern accent—were spot on! And if it weren't for my emulation of Sir Roger Moore's perfect articulation and im-peccable pronunciation of dialogue, I'd be speaking to this day with as southern a twang as Sheriff Pepper's!

That aside, simple *generalizations* aren't necessarily "ste-reotypes" any more than simple preconceptions or *prejudices* about people aren't necessarily "racist" attitudes, which nec-essarily imply presumptions of racial superiority. And simple *bigotry* doesn't necessarily signify racism. So these witless politically correct critics really ought to get both their con-cepts and their misleading terminology straight or shut up!

Then came Sir Roger Moore as James Bond, marking a major milestone in the 007 films by commingling carnally for the very first time with the incredibly comely Bond girl character, Rosie Carver, played by the wholly luscious le-gal secretary–turned Playboy Bunny–turned–blaxploitation actress, Gloria Hendry, who was possessed of the hottest, most provocative pair of womanly thighs ever captured on celluloid.

To this day those same latter–day critics still make much a–to–do about nothing over this supposedly landmark ro-mantically interracial milestone even though manly epic actor, Charlton Heston, beat Bond to the punch a couple years earlier in the apocalyptic sci–fi thriller—the *Omega Man(1971)*—when he took up carnally with the equally alluring black dreadlocks actress, Rosalind Cash, playing an ultimately plague–afflicted, albino mutant sporting an Afro hairstyle and emulating a tough, kick–ass, Pam Grier Mama–style character named Lisa but without the voluptuously protruding bust!

Today the witlessly unthinking politically correct proponents incessantly—and irritatingly—persist in their stupid attempts to co–opt or otherwise rip off as their own supremely apathetic and comatose generation's, all the most positive progress in inter–racial relations actually pioneered and promoted long since by far hipper and cooler generations of youth in times past!

A prime example was when Jordan Charter, in an interview for *Commander Bond.net(CBn)*, asked actress Gloria Hendry this ridiculously contrived and leading question: *"You were the first African-American Bond girl (Unless you count Thumper from Diamonds Are Forever) and at the time it wasn't socially acceptable for a white man to be with a black woman. Do you think that your role in the film helped make the interracial situation more acceptable to audiences?"*—as if it's any more "socially acceptable" now under the supposedly superior "progressive" politically correct regime than it was then in that summer of 1973.

Well, get a clue, Mr. Charter, because that summer when the likes of White House intern Monica Lewinsky was just being born—and decades before she instigated the incredibly insipid "Monicagate" sex scandal by giving United States President Bill Clinton some blow–jobbing head in the Oval Office and West Wing of the White House—I was privately instigating some "socially unacceptable" sex scandal of my own as a lad of *19* in the deep(and supposedly bigoted south) by blissfully coupling with a voluptuous young black woman *13* years my senior named Helen! Now doesn't that just set your pompous, pretentious and not–so–superior politically correct head spinning?

SEXCAPADES

§

Well, on the very same day that I'd performed my car somersault stunt, I did indeed press on to pay an exceptionally cheap fare of $3.65 to ride a *Greyhound* bus from Gulfport, Mississippi to New Orleans, Louisiana to visit at *Loyola University*, situated across St Charles Avenue from Audubon Park, my recently *old* high school sweetheart, Regina, that one last time. Foresightfully enough before leaving I'd locked away in my car trunk my encased trumpet, which I'd carried along expecting to play some songs(like composer Nino Rota's poignant love theme for film director Franco Zeffirelli's *Romeo and Juliet* from 1968)together to Regina's piano accompaniment in one of the airy practice rooms at the university's music college, housed in a quaint old house, as it were, which we'd actually done on my first previous visit there. So at least the crooks at that *B&G Standard Oil* service station were forestalled from looting my trumpet as well as my CB radio and antenna!

And all I got for my trouble was another quick copped feel of Regina's soft and supple little braless breast beneath her rumpled sweat top in her rather snug and cozy dormitory room's bottom bed–bunk—before she put up another of her offputting "wrestling match" struggles as we'd termed them; although our mouths would ache from copious French-kissing. There'd be no *Big Easy* in the *Crescent City*—she wouldn't even invite me to stay overnight after nearly killing myself to visit her—so for another exceptionally cheap fare of $10.95 I rode another *Greyhound* bus from New Orleans, Louisiana back to my hometown of Pensacola, Florida. That would be the absolute last time I would travel to visit Regina.

What Regina had miscalculated were my raging adolescent sexual hormones and the fiery red–hot intense *HOTS* I had to fuck some *forbidden fruit!* After having already slept with my voluptuous Helen I hadn't even been turned on in

33

the slightest by copping another feel of Regina's little breast anyway. And, no, it wasn't a case of the supposed "once–you–go–*black*–you'll–never–go–*back*" mystique either. It was more, rather, a case of once–you–go–**lusty**–you'll–never–go–**runty** again!

Of two honey–pots I would grow demonstrably addicted to in years to come both would be non–black, fairly curvaceous and at least half foreign—the first being Cuban–American, the other being Asian–American.

§

How then did I come to be humping Helen? Well, it was all part and parcel of that hectic, sensational **Live–and–Let–Lie** Summer of 1973—the summer a patent was granted to three inventors for the Automated Teller Machine(ATM)! Instead I was aspiring to become the animated namesake of Jacqueline Susann's best–selling romance novel of 1969, the *"Love Machine!"*

Harking back briefly then: right before the start of my high school year I'd absconded at 17 from a grievous home situation in Pensacola, Florida and went to stay for a short time with the family of my fellow sophomore trumpeter who played(second chair, first section)together with me in our high school band; besides his parents he had two siblings— a younger brother and sister—at their home at 14 Mohawk Trail. Next I passed on to live in roughly the same neighborhood at 109 Tomahawk Trail with another family—whose adopted gay son(who was also a member of my senior class) and younger adopted daughter I'd known and been friends with since the fourth grade in parochial school—throughout our senior year while I'd worked at *Jitney Jungle* and *K–Mart Foods* supermarkets, both a short distance apart on Mobile Highway.

Following our graduation from high school I'd passed

on again to live next throughout the summer of 1972 with my high school band director, his wife and adolescent kids at their home at 306 Washington Street in Gulf Breeze, Florida while I'd worked as a delivery driver for *Fade Auto Parts Co of Brent, Inc* at 105 West Industrial Boulevard, driving to the regular radio tunes of Gilbert O'Sullivan's *"Alone Again(Naturally),"* Elliot Lurie's *"Brandy,"* Elton John's *"Rocket Man,"* and most tediously and redundantly, Eric Clapton's frigging *"Layla."*

In the fall of 1972 I passed on yet again to live at 4400 Fortuna Street with yet another family—whose five kids I'd also known and been friends with since fourth grade in parochial school—throughout my first two semesters attended at *Pensacola Junior College*, working weekends as security guard for the college's privately run *Pensacola Junior College Dormitories* at 1151 College Boulevard. At that time though their eldest son, who'd dropped out of our high school during our senior year to join the United States Army and marry a sweet and tender girl, Joy, I'd introduced him to before then, was away on active service someplace before literally going AWOL at some point.

Then my bastard step–father died of some kind of cancer—ironically as good as a year after he'd summoned me from my senior "Problems of Democracy" class to the high school office to tell me himself by telephone the depressing news that my natural father had died in Boston, Massachusetts. Afterward at the start of the summer of 1973 I actually returned to stay a short time with my negligent mother who'd by then had taken up with a slimy loser of a character named Dale who'd also become her third husband. One late night we both(me and the loser)packed up—fed up—and left at the very same time after I'd intervened physically to prevent them from killing each other in a death struggle over a kitchen steak knife!

After camping out overnight in my car parked on the

street adjacent to *St Stephen Catholic Church* at 900 West Garden Street, I rented the very next day the snug garage room on Whaley Avenue literally less than a neighborhood block away from Regina's family home.

Early on that summer I'd worked part–time along with my high school band director at *Monzingo Music Company*(from which I was buying on installments two brand–new trumpet and flugel horns)at 1410 North Pace Boulevard, apprenticing with him to learn brass musical instrument cleaning and repair.

Later on that summer though I started working for *Tucker Black&White Taxi Inc* at 1019 West Leonard Street, driving a taxicab(city operator permit No 265)during the graveyard shift before being promptly promoted—because of my "clean–cut" looks—to the so–called airport "limousine" shuttle service, driving a glorified passenger van between arriving flights at the *Pensacola Regional Airport*.

On two separate rainy and stormy nights while on the job I'd already luckily escaped other potentially catastrophic vehicular crashes—once on a blindingly torrential trip driving along a dangerously narrow two–lane, two–way road to pick up a special passenger at *Hurlburt Field* Air Force Base bordering Fort Walton Beach, Florida; and once more while transporting a "limousine"–load of passengers along the tortuously winding and slick Bayou Boulevard, turning and twisting its way around *Bayou Texar* when the van abruptly slipped sideways, nearly overturning and putting the interior to deathly silence until I slowed down without braking and recovered complete control of the van. Perhaps I would've done well to carry on my person as my father did a holy card depicting the Apostle St Jude, patron saint of desperate cases and lost causes!   Toward the end of that summer of 1973 I'd met Helen!

§

SEXCAPADES

Apart from enrolling for the first of two sections of the summer session at *Pensacola Junior College* I registered in mid–July at *Skipper's Diving, Inc* on East Wright Street for summer sport scuba diving classes taught by instructor, Dan Stephens.

By roughly mid–August a month later at the height of our training I earned an aspiring superspy's first badge of honor in the form of an unseemly scar resulting from a severe wound suffered in the field of battle. Our instructor dispatched the entire class as combatants to the deep end of our training pool to play a war game dubbed "King of the Bottom of the Pool," wherein the winning object was to be the surviving diver still submerged after forcing all your opponents to surface for air, which could be achieved by one of two methods: ripping off their face mask or cutting off their air supply by turning off their air tank's regulator valve. My most effective strategy was to attack those divers too self–distracted by attacking other opponents. What passed through my mind was composer John Barry's rousing "007 Theme" playing during the climactic underwater battle scene between adverse agents in the James Bond film, *Thunderball(1965)!* When our allotted time was called the upshot was: I'd sure enough stayed submerged at the bottom of the pool after having my own air cut off only once throughout—though I'd managed to both cut off the air and tear off the masks of multiple opponents.

What I hadn't yet noticed—until a fellow learner pointed it out to me afterwards in the locker room by suggesting, "I think you better take a look at your chest!"—I looked at myself in a mirror to discover I'd sustained a severe slash across my upper left chest which opened up like a cleanly and perfectly incised but bloodless eagle's eye! Then I suddenly recalled the sharp, stabbing pain I'd felt by getting caught by a metallic protrusion at the base of another diver's tank when I'd wildly dodged and successfully evaded another opponent's attempted attack. Before long I was prompted to visit the emergency room at *Sacred Heart Hospital* at 5151 North Ninth Avenue to get my incised chest stitched up with sutures!

Two 80–foot sport dives in a splendid coral reef situated off the emerald Gulf Coast and sugary white sandy beaches off the shore of Destin, Florida were the culmination of our scuba class training. Descending the first time had proved to be excruciatingly difficult for me due to an extremely breath–constricting nasal–and–sinus congestion condition, exaggerated by excessive mucus and swollen nasal passages(turbinites)—not to mention a deviated right septum—afflicting me from birth to this day; and unrelieved by the regularly recommended *Drixoral* decongestant pills! As a consequence the head–crushing pressure of going down that anchor rope the first time burst many minute nasal blood vessels, partly filling my face mask with blood. As a fellow diver had put it, I'd taken quite a "beating" over the course of that summer scuba class. My second dive that day went rather swimmingly as well as painlessly. And I became so self–absorbed and rapturously enrapt with the deep diving experience, so to speak, I'd disregarded my air gauge so forgetfully that I was sucking uselessly for air through an all but empty air hose, surfacing hastily on the skimpy surplus of my nearly depleted reserve air supply! Upon finally breaking the surface I found myself remotely separated so far away from my diving party that I had to swim some distance to go back aboard our boat!

Everything was going perfectly well according to plan and right on schedule: without even telling Regina, I'd already arranged with her second best friend, Tina, to drive along with me to the *Pensacola Regional Airport*, drop me off and then drive my car back to my garage–room house, park it on the street—since she lived with her parents only a block over from me in a house at 2222 North Magnolia Street—

and keep my car keys safe for me until I returned from a trip to Boston, Massachusetts to visit my paternal grandmother, Malvina. I recklessly disregarded running the risk of being afflicted with cramps from decompression sickness by flying immediately following two deep–water dives, but since neither dive required decompression upon ascent I chanced it to no ill effect.

Tina was a pretty, golden blond, wavy–haired girl in Regina's high school senior class with a smooth oval face, large eyes, high cheekbones, a straight nose and a full and soft if toothy mouth; and she'd become rather enamored of me after we'd become more closely acquainted. Before I left her at the point of departure I kissed her for the first and last time fully and warmly on her luscious pink lips!

§

A month before at the end of July 1973 a Delta Air Lines Flight 173 DC9–31 aircraft landed about 3000 feet short of Boston's Logan International Airport runway in poor visibility, smashing into a sea wall about 165 feet to the right of the runway and killing aboard all six crew members and 83 passengers—one of the victims dying several months after the tragic accident occurred. At the end of August 1973 then I was boarding a comparable Delta Air Lines aircraft likewise headed for Boston's Logan International Airport. Blessedly the prospect of a catastrophic plane crash would be the last thing preoccupying my mind while seated at a portside window awaiting takeoff! What did arrest my rapt attention nicely was the *tit*illating sight of Helen's bouncy and curvaceous black bosom, fully and softly overflowing her scanty halter top as she moved languidly down the aisle toward me, beaming as she made a direct beeline for the vacant seat next to mine! She flashed her gleaming smile again between her ample lips, softly parted and wet, as she sat right down, rubbing up her smooth bare black shoulder warmly against mine. Her supple breasts bulged partly exposed from her halter top straps! It would be a smoldering hot flight!

This alluring woman introduced herself as proprietor of a beauty salon at 2507 North "E" Street in Pensacola, Florida, handed me her business card, ordered us inflight drinks and invited me to visit her at her studio later on after she returned from Atlanta, Georgia—our transfer stopover point—where she, a former *Ebony* model herself, was attending an *Ebony* fashion show. Naturally I happily accepted her most gracious invitation and indeed pledged myself to pay her an eager visit upon my own return from Boston, Massachusetts!

§

Mine was a rather pensive trip to visit my paternal grandmother, Malvina, at her narrow three–storey row house on sloping White Street in view of Boston Harbor near the airport in East Boston. Principally I'd traveled to Boston to pay my respects at his gravesite in *Holy Cross Cemetery* to my father who'd died of complications related to alcoholism the year before while living and driving himself a taxicab(Hackney Carriage Driver License No 7741)out of Brookline. At my urging my grumpy, crew–cut, white-haired step–grandfather and retired bricklayer, Freddy, led the way to the Roman Catholic *Church of Our Lady of Mt Carmel* on Gove Street in East Boston where I was finally baptized rather late at five years of age.

Also I scouted out on the rather rustic "Heights" of Chestnut Hill the 175–acre, Gothic–built Jesuit campus of *Boston College* to which I'd considered attending myself had any of my paternal relations assisted my relocation. Passing curiously through my mind throughout my lone campus visit were the at once mirthful but melancholic strains to the composition called "Snow Frolic" scored by Francis Lai for the soundtrack to the haunting romantic motion picture drama, *Love Story(1970)*, doubtless due to the proximity of both the film's period and setting at neighboring Harvard University.

Highlighting the trip a comely dark–haired, dark–complexioned young cousin of mine guided me to the breathtaking 50th floor observation deck, dubbed the "Prudential Skywalk," of the 759–foot, glass–and–aluminum *Prudential Tower*—the tallest building outside of New York upon completion in 1964 and still Boston's second–tallest skyscraper after the *John Hancock Tower*(just slightly taller at 788 feet) and still boasting the highest observation deck open to the public in New England! On that rather high note, so to speak, I presently flew back to Pensacola, Florida to keep my fated date with foxy and hot Helen!

§

Sometime that summer following her own high school senior year graduation Regina had come on to me with her crafty overture that we ought to start dating those nebulous "other people," supposedly to appease her parents who were so adamantly opposed to our relationship. It was also her rather lame excuse to exploit the company of another character in her class named Jack to ride his horses—her self–proclaimed uncontrollable "weakness." Regina even contrived to date her best girlfriend's boyfriend so that she, Debra, could in turn date yet another character she was enamored of. Eventually Regina extended her partner–swapping to me and fobbed me off onto her own girlfriend, Debra—a scheme that would badly backfire and go well awry but more in my favor than hers.

For Regina's birthday the spring before I'd spent plenty of time getting better acquainted with Debra when she let me temporarily occupy her free–standing house cottage at 501 West Avery Street to paint(typically to the redundant signature *Morning Has Broken* 8–track cartridge sounds of Cat Stevens)for Regina an oil picture depicting Christ's agony in the garden at Gethsemane—indicative perhaps of the malaise afflicting our relationship—a heartfelt creative gift which Regina ultimately admitted her mother to discard outright(or "throw out" as Regina most euphemistically put it)after being too ashamed and embarrassed to actually display it at her birthday party. This was also about the time that I'd given Regina at her pestering my sublime Henry Mancini–Doc Severinsen collaborative album, *Brass On Ivory(1972)*.

So when Regina's best friend, Debra, finally invited me to accompany her alone one scorching hot summer day to Pensacola Beach, stripping down to her skimpiest string bikini, I was incredibly shocked but scarcely surprised when she initiated a torrid, prolonged, yielding and utterly unresisting make–out session that found us feverishly kissing, caressing, fondling, groping and rolling all over her spread beach blanket for the better part of that sweltering summer afternoon—giving for me new meaning to the term "hot and heavy petting!" I was dripping and Debra was fervidly soft, cuddly and utterly juicy! So I was left both breathless and aghast!

Regina had expressed surprise that I wasn't lonely living my solitary existence in my cloistered little garage space room atop that sloping driveway off Whaley Avenue. It was a snug and cozy little den I'd rented for $10 a week from a kindly German landlady named Anita Utterbach who worked as a prosperous real estate agent and lived with her retired husband and sweet–tempered black cocker spaniel. It was equally divided by an open doorway into just two half sections: one consisted of a twin bed next to a window–facing wooden desk near enough to write at while seated bedside;

the other consisted of a refrigerator, a narrow upright metal shower, a small sink, toilet, wooden wardrobe in which I kept my clothes and footlocker, and a little hot plate. For me it was a supremely peaceful refuge placed in a perfectly pleasant and serene setting where I heard little else in the surrounding neighborhood outside except for the consistently sweet cooing of gentle doves! Gusty and stormy weather occasionally but clamorously walloped the rather flimsy aluminum–roofed structure, hurling brittle tree branches against it, making living there all the more exciting! Most appalling was when late in the middle of the night Anita came barreling up her sloping driveway gunning her massive dark green tank of an *Oldsmobile Cutlass Supreme* luxury car, headlights glaring, braking abruptly and stopping just shy of my doorstep before plowing clear through my wall and into my bed!

At the foot of the bed stood a short wooden bookcase atop which I placed a portable *Admiral* black–and–white television set my father had given me as a childhood gift. Atop a little flat padded armchair by the bed and next to the desk I'd placed my *General Electric* stereo phonograph system with a built–in AM/FM radio which I'd bought with my 1972 federal income tax refund. When I wasn't playing my collection of LP record albums I'd kept the stereo set's FM radio dial set at "Superfidelity" WMEZ("EAZY")94 FM Stereo—the town's sole local easy listening station, which I'd grown so sentimentally fond of listening to, most especially late at night, ever since my long–time gay boyhood friend, John, with whom I'd roomed throughout our high school senior year, had softly set his nightstand clock radio to elegant "EZ" for us to fall asleep to each and every night. Its display dial glowed, shedding a soothing blue light that comforted me throughout the quiet night.

No, I've never heard such magnificent and richly moving music playing in either elevators or doctors' offices so I've never unduly denigrated it as such either. And I soundly disregard all those disparaging out of sheer ignorance and punky stupidity what should if anything be labeled simply **orchestral** music, which is exactly what it is; so I make no apologies to anyone for loving easy listening!

For the preceding couple of years I'd been compelled by happenstance to live under the albeit charitable roofs—as well as the decidedly well–regulated and orderly household rules—of four different families. Suddenly I was then foot-loose and fancy–free, and finally liberated and fully exempt from anybody else's arbitrary, capricious and conformist rules and regulations. I was once and for all perfectly free and unfettered to come and go and do precisely whatever, whenever, wherever and however I pleased! And that was as incredibly and supremely refreshing as it was liberating!

So then I profoundly reveled in listening to heart–and–soul–stirring EZ music—or for that matter jazz trum-peter Maynard Ferguson powerfully wailing "Hey Jude," "MacArthur Park" or "Round Midnight" or legendary singer Barbra Streisand flawlessly phrasing her mellowest and most moving melodies on "The Way We Were"(her two–time platinum album, not the movie)—at anytime and at any damn hour of the night or day or *ALL* night if I damn well felt like it! Suffice it to say then: I was wallowing *ecstatically* in my new–found freedom and was anything and everything *but* lonely—especially since I ventured there in inviting over my first overnight feminine guests!

After all, that year I'd already adopted Barry White's *Love Unlimited Orchestra*'s romantically moving and velvety smooth *Love's Theme(1973)*as my amorous spirit's signature song!

One of my more womanly maiden voyagers, as it were, was a curvaceous and voluptuous young blond waitress named Nancy whom I'd met while she was working at an all–night *Coffee Cup* restaurant on Cervantes Street I'd fre-quented for breakfast following my graveyard shift driving the taxicab. She once accompanied me on a date to the local gay musical revue club called the *Yum Yum Tree*, where I must modestly and humbly boast that I attracted much more erotic attention from the club's lip–syncing transvestite performers, stopping by in turn to sit down at our booth to overtly and playfully flirt with me, until I was flushed with blushing embarrassment. All Nancy would be flushed with was redness from overindulgent drinking to mighty excess!

She readily returned with me to my cramped room and splayed herself out upon my twin bed with utter squirming abandon. And I wallowed swimmingly in kissing her full luscious lips, her hot breath reeking of alcohol, and caressing her full fleshy bosom once I peeled off her bra. But by the time I got round with breathlessly bated breath to anxiously unzip the front of her extremely snug and tight–fitting corduroys, exposing to sight and touch her softly plump paunch, she'd already passed out cold from heady drunkenness. Now I could've easily exploited Nancy's incapacitated condition, and taken full sexual advantage of this undoubtedly lush and overflowing girl, but my remaining gentlemanly scruples prevented me. So we simply fell peacefully asleep, snug and warm in each other's arms until the morning, she leaving me her heavily–buckled belt as a consoling souvenir of our memorable if somewhat innocent and virtuous night together.

Sometime that summer I'd literally swept another petite blond waitress with pale but perky little tits named Jan off her feet, carrying her in broad daylight into the airy bedroom of her beach cottage to screw; she was squirming wet but once she got her bra stripped off she freaked out and abruptly copped out, complaining that the action we were getting on together was coming a little too fast.

§

At Helen's provocation I'd effortlessly overlook all my remaining gentlemanly scruples!

I drove over slickly dressed to Helen's beauty salon and studio on North "E" Street promptly for our date. Directly she closed up her shop and invited me to accompany her to her private residence—a humble mobile home immovably parked in the rear of her property.

To the right of her entrance I noticed right off that her trailer front contained a confined but open bedroom containing a rather big and inviting bed. Helen presently seated me on her cushiony living room sofa situated along the wall of that front bedroom. Following some perfunctory if hospitable niceties she served me at least two brimming tumblerfuls of red wine. She wanted me either drunk or relaxed or both; so I accommodated her so long as she was swilling along with me, which she was! Before long she politely excused herself to the rear of her trailer to slip into something more comfortable and soon reemerged wearing absolutely nothing but exceptionally transparent beige lingerie, displaying every sleek curve and bulge of her incredibly ample but well proportioned shape. Her exceptionally soft and supple breasts and swollen nipples poked proudly out of her flimsy see–through nightie. Her look was powerfully seductive as she sat down alongside me, folding me warmly in her arms, and I knew for sure that I was just about to get laid right then and there for the very first time! And that it was going to be *real* good—and it was!

Before long—in the fever heat of making out and feeling each other up on Helen's sofa—she pulled my phallus out of my pants, clenching it, and had a firm hold on its neck as it stood bolt upright from her grip, throbbing a strong eight inches long.

"Shall we move someplace more comfortable?" I asked her mischievously.

"*You're* the man!" she chided me with a wry, frowning

face.

So as any *man* would do, supposedly, I picked up Helen bodily, wobbled with her but a step to that front room before plunking her down onto the bed and hastily stripping off her satiny nightie and panties, collapsing atop her. Warmly embracing, kissing, and caressing, I wallowed in her supremely silky breasts pressing up against my own soft chest from beneath. I was sprawled between her tender and thickset thighs and, strongly aroused, smoothly penetrated her luscious pussy with my erect and hard prong.

"This is your first time, isn't it?" she asked me with a knowing whisper.

"Yes," I admitted grudgingly, all bravado gone and abruptly replaced with something more akin to affection.

She grew more miserly with her kisses as she tugged greedily to incite me to start thrusting into her, undulating rhythmically underneath me. Since I'd never even jacked myself off before in my whole life—and still haven't—I didn't really know quite what to expect. Rather than lunge and plunge as I would come to do with so many others in so many times to come, I instinctively pressed the mound of my pelvis firmly against hers, grindingly rubbing down on her the harder and longer I grew inside of her. She felt intensely hot, engulfing me with her warm wetness, but I was actually wondering whether that was all there was to it—when that rushing, dizzying blindness of overwhelming orgasm clouded over my eyesight!

"Oh! Ah, yes," I thought to myself at the startling revelation, so heady and mind–blowing. "I *see* now!"

So I would go to Helen to sleep with her a lot more so many times before it was all over—especially when I was so desperately hard up and horny that I couldn't stand it until I was lying between her spreadeagled legs and fucking her again! And she'd let me!

At home back in bed in my dark minuscule room I would

come all over myself, staining my bedsheets, simply by rubbing my cocked dick hard against my mounted mattress, thinking about her all the while—the closest I ever came to manual masturbation! Sleep?! What a contradiction in terms? Whoever heard of sleeping while fucking? Sleepily fucking—perhaps! Well, thanks to Helen and her liberal—and luscious—initiation to sex and screwing I was habitually addicted and hooked on fucking big–time, always and forevermore!

That was late August 1973. But before we were through by early February 1974, Helen had rather turned the sexual tables on herself for she'd grown fonder and had fallen somewhat in love with me. So much so that the very night before I was appointed to travel and overturn my car visiting Regina at *Loyola University* in New Orleans, Helen had called me in tears, crying uncontrollably aloud, pledging her love for me and pleading with me to come over and be with her.

"I want to *marry* you!" she bawled lustily. Much to my everlasting shame and sorrow, I most apologetically and ashamedly refused, being too immature and inexperienced to know how to rightly react.

Wherever you are, my dearly beloved Helen, I most humbly and contritely apologize and beg your pardon. I so selfishly abandoned you in your most trying time of need, pandering to the malicious chicanery of a puerile, punk little girl, who only pretended to love me, instead of rightly going to you. And for that I'm truly, sincerely and forever very, very sorry. If I could turn back time, I promise you, I would've done things altogether differently, answering your emotional summons by putting myself at your complete disposal!

§

READ THE SIGNS:
Admonitions to Men

SEXCAPADES

Appraise the appropriateness and compatibility of any prospective romantic partner by appreciating the maturity (or immaturity) of their aesthetic tastes and sensibilities.

Regina was an extremely immature little girl who pestered me no end to acquire for her pop culture books the likes of Erich Fromm's *The Art of Loving* and Alvin Toffler's *Future Shock.* She thought libertarian film actor and card–carrying *National Rifle Association(**NRA**)*member, Kurt Russell, was a romantic heartthrob! Why, she even thought that California Secretary of State(1971–1975)and future California "Governor Moonbeam"–to be(1975–1983), Edmund Gerald "Jerry" Brown Jr, would ultimately become President of the United States of America! Read the signs then, my friends! I failed to read the signs and it cost me dearly the love of my first really good woman! Don't make the same lamentable and mournful mistake! Read the signs!

TWO:
THE MAN WITH THE GOLDEN PUN

*"I can't believe anyone mistook you for an Iranian—who would believe you are anyone else but 'my good pen pal,' a super Italian lover, who doesn't dance too badly either! Watch out!!!"—**Lyn, 20 January 1975***

T<i>he Man with the Golden Gun(1974)</i>, despite Sir Roger Moore's second *Saint*–like cool but often–times tougher and harder–edged portrayal of not–so–secret British agent James Bond 007, was, except perhaps for his seventh outing in *A View To A Kill(1985)*, the piss–poorest and lame–assest of the **EON** productions he participated in, with an absurdly preposterous and plot–less story lamely trying to trade on its timely link to the so–called "energy crisis" of the period. Now how flat is that?

Besides bikini–clad Swedish actress Britt Ekland, the flick's endowed with few redeeming features—like its title tune theme sung by Scottish singer, Lulu, with her lusty melisma style, but which even superlative composer, John Barry, has more recently complained was his least favorite Bond theme composition. For me it was a hauntingly melancholic theme unbefitting the flick's frivolity and name–checking James Bond, which even my own bitch of a mother when I played it once on her home stereo asked, aghast, why I liked such incredibly sad music. Why, even the latter–day critics have harpingly whined about the flick's supposedly "sexist" tone in its depiction of Britt Ekland's "Mary Goodnight" character as a supposedly stereotypical blond bimbo—as if each and every "Bond girl," so–called, has to be a feminist–championing "equal" to Bond in each and every impossibly contrived scenario. Well, it's that type of politically correct, wistful, wishful thinking mentality that's pretty much ruined the original spontaneous creativity of the series. Suffice it to say, this particular entry was for the most part just plain silly and stupid and Sir Roger Moore easily out–classed the script material he was given to work with!

Calcutta–born Marne Maitland(Lazar)made impressive appearances in *Hammer Horror's The Terror of the Tongs(1961)* as the beggar, *Phantom of the Opera(1962)*as Xavier and *The Reptile(1966)*as the Malay.

James Cossins(Colthrope)likewise appeared memorably as the Seagull Island coroner in *The Deadly Bees(1967)*as well as in *Hammer Horror's The Lost Continent(1968)*as chief engineer Nick, *The Horror of Frankenstein(1970)*as Dean, *Blood From The Mummy's Tomb(1971)*as the elder male nurse, along with *Fear In The Night(1972)*as the Doctor; just as Michael Goodliffe(Bill Tanner)played Professor Jules Heitz in *Hammer Horror's The Gorgon(1964)*.

§

With the *Universal Product Code(**UPC**)*symbol being scanned commercially for the very first time in late June— on a pack of *Wrigley's* chewing gum at the *Marsh* supermarket in Troy, Ohio no less!—1974 headed the decade for a bad period all around.

As an aspiring superspy all of 20 still enrolled full–time at *Pensacola Junior College* I'd gotten wind of a former spook from the "Company" or the "Agency"—or "Other Government Agency" otherwise known as the *Central Intelligence Agency*(quite a contradiction in terms itself!)— named Robert R Musselwhite(dubbed "Musselhead" by an administrative colleague)who was actually employed as Dean of the so–called "Evening College." So I went to his second–floor administration building office to meet, visit and ultimately befriend this character—a tallish, slim, rather elegant, deep–voiced, white–haired, well–spoken gentleman who smoked dark brown pencil–thin cigarettes and fancied himself a lookalike–with–hair of actor *Telly Savalas!* He was in fact a dead ringer for deceased actor, *Richard Devon*, who specialized in playing gangsters on television serials.

Presently we formed something of a mutually symbiotic relationship: I grilled him for intriguing anecdotes about superspy exploits; he stroked his own already over–inflated, ego–tripping mussel–head to deign to condescend to talk down to discourse, lecture and preach to whom he presumed was an awestruck youth. Our overlong conversations helped him at that to pass the time, which apparently he had a lot of on his hands to spare, especially once his hot and foxy, black–haired, heavily–rouged, full–figured Italian secretary named Carol left for the night. So to extend our discussions until his exit at ten o'clock he'd frequently invite me to join him for dinner, driving us in his economy car—a fiery red *American Motor Company(AMC)*compact hatchback *Gremlin*, ironically enough!—to a homey booth diner on East Cervantes Street called *Jerry's Drive–In*, prominently displaying in years to come on a wooden wall that infamous red–swimsuit–Farrah Fawcett poster, which served up the most scrumptious open–bun barbeque plate ever tasted!

A rabid booster of President Richard M Nixon, this spook character, much like then Secretary of State Henry Kissinger, who'd proclaim rather gratuitously that history would relegate "Watergate" to a minor footnote, likewise labeled the national scandal a "trifle!"

Well, even I was personally beholden to *anomalous* President Nixon, whom I was grateful to for taking the extremely unconventional and unconservative step of indexing Social Security for inflation, which was invaluable to a struggling student such as myself receiving a paltry monthly death benefit from my deceased father's Social Security funds until I was 22 years of age so long as I stayed in school full–time! President Nixon even established Supplemental Security Income(SSI)—unlike supposedly populist President William Jefferson "Bill" Clinton who roughly 22 years later in February 1996 would effectively end welfare entitlement in America!

Towing the classically knee–jerk "national security" line, this spook character, Mr Musselhead, boasted how he'd witnessed spook administrators such as himself, admitting that he'd never himself worked as a "field agent" operative, would tear up and defiantly ignore presidential executive orders, presumably those prohibiting domestic spying activities against American citizens or political assassinations of foreign leaders and heads of state; for Mr Musselhead was most fervently all in favor of such illegal criminal acts committed as the violent overthrows of legitimate elected governments abroad and their permanent replacement by puppet dictators, despots and regimes partial to America's "vital interests" overseas: expanding multi–national corporate interests, exploiting the natural resources and forcibly imposing America–brand democracy in unsuspecting countries all around the world. "I *approve* of that!" he'd pompously proclaim—as if anybody gave a damn about what he approved of! In fact, he'd belittle field agents as those placed lowest on the proverbial covert intelligence totem pole! Little wonder one of his favorite expressions was, "Hell's Bells!"

Once on a smaller scale he even extended his deceptive and surreptitious hegemonic–minded, meddlesome interference to me by outright lying, telling me falsely that an office secretary in the building who'd been typing–for–pay some short stories of mine was wondering where her payment was, when with truth she'd expressed absolutely no such apprehension.

Well, I'd returned the embarrassment in kind: sometimes Mr Musselhead would invite me to accompany him to a closet employee break–room for a small Styrofoam cup of coffee. And once when some frustrated and petty biddy who observed me taking a Styrofoam cup of break–room coffee without his attendance went whining in protest to Mr Musselhead, I proceeded then to march across the avenue to the nearest supermarket to purchase the largest can of *Maxwell House* ground coffee from the shelf that I could find, returning to present it in person to the biddy at her counter service station with my smiling compliments!

Sometime during my visits to Mr Musselhead then a full–

fleshed, full–lipped, dark–haired, large–eyed young student assistant in his office named Kathy took a shine to me and eventually accompanied me one night on Whaley Avenue in *East Hill* to my snug garage room, where I'd banged her hard in the bed, making her cry out aloud, banging the bed headboard hard and noisily into the wall! What had really gotten me turned on were her rather bloated but unforgettably bullet–shaped breasts that had burst out into full view once I'd hastily stripped off her top. Hers was only the second pussy I'd ever pumped but in a letter she wrote me in January 1975 she'd confided then that her "first interest(in me)had been satisfied." Well, that went likewise for the two of us and my superspy sexploits career was off to a fantastic, killer–diller start!

§

During the first section of summer term 1974 at *Pensacola Junior College* I was provocatively confronted with yet another scanty halter top overflowing with full and fleshy feminine breasts once more in the shape of a voluptuous, full–mouthed, big–eyed brunet and 28–year–old secretary for the college's dental hygiene department named Jean who was an actress Janet Leigh–lookalike, and whom I met ironically enough in an evening "general *biology*" class no less! Now it gets no more erotically portentous than that!

With Jean I'd stay for roughly the next four years in a relatively stable and steady romantic—and frequently sexually active—relationship from which I'd actually stray and betray her relatively little over that time, cheating on her only infrequently until I would ultimately(and *stupidly*)jilt her to marry in June 1978 a crazed 22–year–old Cuban–American chick from Key West, Florida—the first(and worst)profoundly(and supremely)**stupid** mistake of my entire life bar none! In the interim I would occasionally overindulge and plunge into carnal dissipation by pumping some strange pussy!

For the first time I two–timed Jean two times with a vivacious, mischievously–smiling and rather racy young brunet named Lyn whom I first met while she was working part–time as a sales clerk in the *Montgomery Ward*(before it became known as *Wards*)department store at suburban *Cordova Mall*. Later on she'd work in varying capacities over the years as a secretary. Lyn was a bit of a bawdy babe and reminded me something of actress Elizabeth Ashley, who originally was herself a Floridian born in Ocala. But right off we hit it off, and the first time we heatedly made out once we parked in the mall lot after she drove me in her car to mine, and we were swapping spit and tongues, she was gripping my dripping dick through my wet pants—making a most lasting memorable impression!

Twice we got it on though the first time—at her *Cordova Regency* apartment on Bayou Boulevard—I nearly didn't get off at first, experiencing my first bout with sexual dysfunction, so–called, out of my admitted guilt for two–timing Jean. But Lyn was politely patient, I excused myself to take a quick warm shower in her bathtub and directly we got down and dirty! I had no particular motive for two–timing Jean except for being young and lusting to explore more of the feminine sex. And Lyn was exceedingly sexy, seductive and gowned herself in lacy see–through lingerie from which the thick dark nipples of her firm and perky breasts protruded prominently, inviting hearty fondling and sucking. So when we heatedly got it on again together sometime later on at her upstairs townhouse bedroom on tree–lined North 15th Avenue in *East Hill*, both my sexual guilt and dysfunction had proved to be quite short–lived and not at all a...*short-fall!* Quite the contrary, Lyn wasn't just a little disappointed and upset when I'd declined to stay overnight after our second tryst. Nevertheless we remained faithful friends and pen pals—even after she got married with children in early

December 1976—until we lost touch altogether by the early 1980s. Before then though my superspy sexploits would take me across the state of Florida and into new and uncharted erotic territory.

THREE:
THE GUY WHO LOVED ME

*"I miss you and I'll be really glad to see you when you come home in June."—**Anne, 12 April 1977***

The Spy Who Loved Me(1977)continued the sorry and disturbing trend—started with *You Only Live Twice(1967)*, most aptly scripted by children's book writer, Roald Dahl—of deviating grossly and drastically from Ian Fleming's original source novel material, degrading and reducing the Bond saga to cartoonish if spectacular comic strip camp! Small wonder that English director Lewis Gilbert would carry on his extravagantly campy Bond trilogy full circle with *Moonraker(1979)*.

The Spy Who Loved Me was simply the camp of *You Only Live Twice* revamped with nuclear ballistic missile submarines instead of manned spacecraft capsules being hijacked by nefarious villains! It likewise continued the equally sorry trend starting with "Nick Nack" in *The Man With The Golden Gun* of casting ridiculously cornball characters like "Jaws." Apart from Sir Roger Moore's consistently *Saint*-like cool and sophisticated performance as not–so–secret British agent James Bond 007 and Carly Simon's title theme song(*"Nobody Does It Better"*), the flick boasts few redeeming features except for a couple of exceptionally striking and stunning "Bond girls"—neither of whom were the powerfully bland Barbara Bach: both the breathtaking, incredibly leggy Caroline Munro("Naomi")and the sublime, incredibly busty Valerie Leon(Sardinian hotel receptionist), being five-foot–eight and five–foot–eleven respectively, were the two true, *sauciest* treats of that flick!

George Baker(Captain Benson)appeared notably as Martin Delambre in *Curse of the Fly(1965)*, an uncredited NASA Engineer in *You Only Live Twice(1967)*and most memorably as Sir Hilary Bray in *On Her Majesty's Secret Service(1969)*.

Edward de Souza(Sheikh Hosein)deftly played charming characters in *Hammer Horror's Phantom of the Opera(1962)* as Harry Hunter and *Kiss of the Vampire(1963)*as Gerald Harcourt.

Vernon Dobtcheff(Max Kalba)appeared notably as Sir Bernard Newsmith in the British horror flick, *The Beast in the Cellar(1970)*.

Gorgeous Miss World(1969), Eva Reuber-Staier would reprise her role of Rublevitch in both *For Your Eyes Only(1981)* and *Octopussy(1983)*.

Robert Brown(Admiral Hargreaves)appeared notably as a guard in Roger Corman's collaboration with the incomparable Vincent Price in *Masque of the Red Death(1964)* as well as playing parts in *Hammer Horror's The Abominable Snowman(1957)*as Ed Shelley and Raquel Welch's *One Million Years BC(1966)*as Akhoba before becoming "M" in the James Bond films, 1983-1989.

Milton Reid(Sandor)excelled at expertly playing menacing bald ogres in *Blood of the Vampire(1958)*as the executioner, *Hammer Horror's The Terror of the Tongs(1961)*as an uncredited Tong guardian, *Dr No(1962)*as Dr No's guard, *Casino Royale(1967)*as a Temple guard, *Blood on Satan's Claw (1971)* as a dog handler and Vincent Price's lackluster *Dr Phibes Rises Again(1972)*as Biederbeck's ill–fated manservant.

Cyril Shaps(Dr Bechmann)appeared most notably but uncredited in *Hammer Horror's The Terror of the Tongs (1961)* and *Rasputin the Mad Monk(1966)*as Foxy Face.

Sri Lankan Albert Moses(Barman)had already appeared alongside Sean Connery as Ghulam in *The Man Who Would Be King(1975)*before reappearing in another Bond film as Sadruddin in *Octopussy(1983)*.

Shane Rimmer(Commander Carter)appeared uncredited yet quite credit–worthy in the Bond films *You Only Live Twice(1967)*as the Hawaii Radar Operator and *Diamonds Are Forever(1971)*as Tom.

George Roubicek(Stromberg One Captain)had already appeared notably as an American Spacecraft #2 Astronaut in *You Only Live Twice(1967)*.

Victor Tourjansky(man with the bottle)would be

back, wielding more deadly beverage containers in both *Moonraker(1979)*as another man with the bottle and *For Your Eyes Only(1981)*as the man with the wine glass!

Film composer Marvin Hamlisch's often disco–oriented soundtrack for the flick further signaled and reflected the continued downslide of the decade as a whole. Going from worsted double–breasted suits by Saville Row to bell–bottom pants and wing–collared print shirts, the decade went from classy to cheesy in the relatively short span of ten years! It would also represent the lowest point in the life of an aspiring superspy, who'd hit rock bottom hard and find himself at his lowest ebb ever.

§

Following my graduation from *Pensacola Junior College* in June 1974 with an Associate of Arts(AA)degree I took the next fall semester off before matriculating—at the influential behest of Mr Musselhead—to the prestigious *George Washington University(GWU)*in Washington, DC—fondly known then as the *"Tel Aviv of the Potomac"*—to enroll in its School of Government and Business for the winter 1975 semester. Financially I couldn't afford to stay and keep up paying its exorbitant tuition fees without plunging deeper into exorbitant debt, but in my single semester there I at least distinguished myself by being awarded the School of Arts and Sciences *Alexander Wilbourne Weddell Prize* for writing the best essay on "spreading peace among the nations of the world," being the sole junior so honored at senior commencement exercises held at the *Daughters of the American Revolution(DAR)Constitution Hall* on Northwest "D" Street that spring of 1975.

Apart from a couple heated make–out sessions with a couple hot–and–bothered young co–ed chicks at different times I studied seriously and did no sexual gallivanting until Jean arrived to stay with me for the week–long semester spring break when we holed up in a downtown hotel for a prolonged and strenuous conjugal visit! I was being loyal and faithful to Jean—in my aspiring superspy's fashion.

Following an informal evening dance–social in the lobby piano room lounge(where students would often delight in listening to me play on my trumpet Burt Bacharach's pretty pop tune from 1967's *Casino Royale, The Look of Love!*)at GWU's Thurston Hall dormitory building on Northwest "F" Street a cute petite chick from Lowell, Massachusetts named Robin accompanied me back to my snug and warm seventh floor room(756)at the downtown YMCA at 1736 "G" Street, NW; but once she got down to getting her perky little tittie groped she got too itchy and thought better of it to go.

From my trumpet practice in that piano room lounge I was recruited by its director to play in his pep band for the *George Washington Colonials* basketball team during their Friday night games—to which we commuted across the Potomac River bridge in a battered bus and at which I played 1st trumpet for their *"Buff And Blue"* theme song!

During my short single–semester stay at GWU I was likewise privileged to walk to attend at least three superb performances at the *John F Kennedy Center for the Performing Arts*(on the building itself titled the *John F Kennedy Memorial Center for the Performing Arts* and commonly referred to simply as the *Kennedy Center*)situated on the Potomac River adjacent to the infamous *Watergate* apartment complex. That performing arts center had opened on 8 September 1971—less than four years before my own arrival in DC.

For my birthday Friday the 24th of January 1975 I attended a wonderful recital played by Brooklyn, NY–born pianist, **Peter Nero**, at the center's 2400–seat Concert Hall; most notably for me **Peter Nero** played the million–seller single rendition of the *Summer of '42* film love theme!

At the center's 2300–seat Opera House I attended equally memorable performances put on by famed French mime artist, **Marcel Marceau**, as well as celebrated *King–and–I* actor, **Yul Brynner**, playing in *Love Story* **Erich Segal**'s musical play, *Odyssey!*

On another night a chubby blond chick waved me over to visit from the open window of her room overlooking the shared sunken alley separating our directly facing wings in the old faded red–brick building.

Student housing was so scarce that the university leased out several floors of the YMCA to rent at marked up prices to students desperate to cohabit communally. Fortunately I'd secured a private room of my own directly from the YMCA management.

Apparently anxious to get us alone and on our own—and me to herself—she hastily chased her several female "suite–mates" out of that corner room at the end of the wing hall. She was possessed of an exceptionally pretty, flawlessly soft and smooth face, sparkling eyes and full luscious lips. She wore a jeans jump–suit, her curvaceous breasts bursting out from her flimsy soft white top to be groped and fondled at will as she squirmed tortuously beneath me, pleading unspokenly to be mounted and fucked—which I was at once both inclined and reluctant to do until her roommates finally broke in upon us impatient to return. That chubby chick had been impetuously hot and wet and one I really regret having let get away!

Going back to Pensacola, Florida for further summer semester study at *Pensacola Junior College* I decided to remain and register at the local upper–level *University of West*(or **WORST** as it's more fondly known)*Florida(UWF)*from which I graduated in mid–December 1976 with my first worthless bachelor of arts(BA)degree in criminal justice.

Jean, whom I'd encouraged to return to school had herself graduated Phi Theta Kappa from the junior college and prepared to transfer on scholarship to *Florida Atlantic*

*University(FAU)*in Boca Raton. We'd been cohabiting together, shacked up at three different places in the meantime, but by January 1977 we'd separated and I was temporarily left behind living alone in our shared cinder block cottage on the more impoverished west side of town. I was awaiting transfer to the very same university in March 1977 pending arrangements to register for graduate study in secondary education and political science. During that short separation was when I met a man–eating nymphomaniac named Anne!

§

One fated night—the first and last throughout that rather wretched and cold winter term apart—I ventured over for nostalgia's sake to my favorite *East Hill* side of town to a flashy and noisy new discotheque at *Cordova Mall* named "*Big Daddy's*," brilliantly ablaze with pulsating strobe lights above and kaleidoscopic colors shedding fitful and erratic beams from beneath the transparent dance floor below.

Now I've always richly amused myself at bars by observing many a loser of a bloke(or dude)looking to score by approaching indiscriminately many a bird(or chick)with worn–out come–ons doomed to fail—in the forlorn hope that the sexual law of averages would ultimately work in his favor, which usually never pans out—only to get blown off with a rude rejection. One thing I've learned from women over the years is that if and when they're at all really interested in you—sexually or otherwise—then they'll usually let you know it in quite straightforward terms! And if and when they're not interested in you then all the hackneyed come–ons in the world won't bring you any closer to getting laid much less getting laid good. So take a practical tip and you'll be way ahead of the game: look attentively for the chick who already has her eye intently on you and then make your move! That's precisely how I played meeting that night a pair of foxy young fillies named Olivia Anne and Christina—Anne and Chris for short—a red–hot blond–and–brunet duo all ready to get down!

It was Anne, a perfectly busty and lusty blond, who'd had her rapt eye on me. And it was Anne who'd invited me out that very night, treating me to a big breakfast at the nearest all–night diner right after the disco's closing at two o'clock in the morning. And it was Anne who'd driven me that very night to her shared house at 555 Navy Boulevard, apologetically laying me down on some low–level bedding on their wooden living room floor since her roomie, Chris, occupied their bedroom, and then proceeded to fuck me wildly and wantonly into the early morning, making a special point to actually *time* by her little portable clock how *many* times—*six* all told—she could make me get off within one *half* hour by alternately sucking and fucking my already tuckered out dick! Even for an aspiring superspy of just 22 that excessively orgasmic but steamy ejaculating session had worn both it—and me—well out! Finally I simply collapsed, my deadened dick benumbed with aching pain, wondering whether I'd be paralyzed for life from the waist down! And at the disco earlier I hadn't bought that chick even the first drink, so go figure!

Later on one afternoon, Chris, a slimmer, taller but shapely and admittedly prettier brunet paid me a lone visit to my wretched cottage and acted provocatively receptive to letting me get into her hot and wet pants, freely perching and necking on my bed, but once she let her perfectly perky and thickly nippled breasts burst out to be caressed, kissed and sucked she thought better of it—perhaps out of guilt from interloping upon her best friend and roomie's fresh sexual turf—and abruptly broke off from going all the way. Then she proceeded to report back on our carnal encounter to Anne, who promptly came over to confront me with a rather prematurely possessive attitude about my "making a pass" at poor innocent and helpless Chris, who'd freely climbed top-less into my bed.

Perhaps in retrospect I'd been put within some womanly early–warning system to some two–timing test, who knows for sure?! Nevertheless I parted on fantastic terms with amorous Anne, who turned out to be an artistic designer of custom–made–polished–and–painted fake fingernails, and for a time we kept up a long–distance correspondence with one another.

§

Following my transfer on Jean's heels to *Florida Atlantic University(FAU)*in Boca Raton, Florida—reputedly the spam capital of the world—my extracurricular superspy sexploits somewhat fizzled out for a short time except for a couple of fleeting erotic encounters early on—one with a rather raunchy and confused 29–year–old Jewish floozy named Jemell still baffled about what course to take in life. She came onto me strong from the start and my sole excuse for doing her was because she was an incredibly easy but not altogether unsavory lay. A little petite but still shapely and supple her most enticing feature was her satiny soft and burnished skin; she possessed rather tempting pouty lips too. And when the time came to actually do the nasty she herself came readily attired in some pinkish flimsy lingerie with her tight but pudgy little pussy brimming with peachy wetness. In her springy twin dormitory bed I did her good, turning her bawdy bravado into some semblance of softly affection-ate and gentle contentment. And that amply surprised me and made me slightly reluctant to leave her alone as hastily as I did.

If GWU in DC was supposed to be the "Tel Aviv of the Potomac" then FAU in Boca Raton("Mouse Mouth"), Florida should well have been the "Tel Aviv of the south" since it appeared to be profusely populated by an overabundance of hot and tender Jewish co–ed chicks on the make(over 15 percent of the population is Jewish making the town one of the nation's teeming Jewish communities)! One of them was a decidedly handsome, well–made and remarkably warm and bosomy young Italian named Emmy possessed of raven-black hair, large eyes, luscious lips, mightily thickset thighs and, much like Jemell, silky smooth skin which looked emblazoned with bronze.

For Emmy my throbbing rock–hard rod would shoot straight out bolt upright at the sheer sight of her striking nakedness, but when confronted with actually penetrating her honeyed wetness my burning, overwrought dick would ejaculate and shoot off prematurely each and every time with overanxious anticipation—much to the bitter disappointment and frustration of us both. Sympathetic and patient throughout, Emmy would caressingly grasp my rigidly erect dick once it cocked up with both her hands, conspicuously pleased if not amused by the firm hold she had on my uncontrollably misfiring love muscle!

Amidst two separate abortive attempts at proper and deep penetration I got unduly distracted but completely captivated—heart and soul—in June 1977 by a young virginal but completely, cold–bloodedly crazed, 22–year–old, Auburn–haired Cuban–American chick named Elizabeth, whom I could not only controllably and forcefully fuck to my heart's content but whom by June 1978 would become my first most fiendish and demonic shrew of a wife—and whom until(and even beyond)our blessed and most heavenly divorce on *9 April 1981* made my youthful life a wholly unmitigated and miserable hell on earth!

"Good luck with it," the Escambia County sheriff's deputy process server bid me gladly Wednesday the 8th of October 1980 once he delivered to me my first divorce papers at my private dorm room at UWF campus.

DICKY GALORE

To this day I celebrate that infinitely appreciated, heaven–sent *final* divorce date as an international holiday I pridefully title: *Liberation From All Wickedly Evil, Inhuman And Malevolent Bitches Day!*

§

READ THE SIGNS:
Admonitions to Men

Appraise the appropriateness and compatibility of any prospective romantic partner by appreciating the maturity(or immaturity)of their aesthetic tastes and sensibilities.

Elizabeth to this day was and is the most immature, childishly contrary and infantile punk harpy I've ever met or encountered in my entire life! An avowed atheist she idolized not God but anything and everything about the outright tackiest decade of the 20th Century: the 1970s! She thought TV actors *Patrick Duffy*(of *Man From Atlantis, Dallas*), scientologist *John(**Revolta**)Travolta*(of *Welcome Back Kotter*)and alcoholic, *"Baby–Come–Back"*–crooning *David Soul*(of *Starsky and Hutch*)were the living limits of romantic heartthrobs. She thought the noisy racket of *Abba*, the *Bee Gees* and Miami–spawned *KC&The Sunshine Band*—and not to forget oftentimes soppy, song–mumbler *Neil Diamond*—embodied the ultimate musical experience. She thought the sole movies of the century consisted of the extremely over–rated *Saturday Night Fever(1977)*—a film farsightedly *banned* in Malaysia—and the tawdry *American Gigolo(1980)*starring Richard Gere as the most improbable male prostitute ever conceived! Reputable "Superman" actor Christopher Reeve himself intrepidly rejected the gigolo role as "distasteful." *Chicago's* self–destructive breakup number—*"If You Leave Me Now"*—suited Elizabeth perfectly as her quintessential

72

signature theme song.

She got turned on most by that incredibly charming Luke–rapes(seduces?)–and–then–marries–Laura–to–white-wash–the–rape soap opera saga on ABC TV's *General Hospital.*

In a most bizarre twist to Elizabeth's mentally deranged immaturity she admitted to actually stalking to his house an FAU mathematics instructor simply because he supposedly resembled in appearance(he didn't)alcoholic actor David Soul whom she was really so fanatically infatuated and ob-sessed with !

A sage word to the wise to all aspiring superspies: *Read the bleedin'* **SIGNS!**

FOUR:
MOONMAKER

*"You are a **very special** friend. It's funny, even if you don't keep in touch with someone, sometimes things may happen that remind you of that person. So, I guess that 'out–of–sight' doesn't necessarily mean 'out–of–mind'!"—**Rena, 31 December 1981**

Moonraker(1979)might very well have been re-titled *James Bond Goes Into Orbit!* Well, why not? The Three Stooges went into orbit in 1962—albeit with far funnier and more entertaining effects! Cashing in on exploiting the inexplicable popularity of that asininely adolescent *Star Wars* saga, 007's outer space caper was just about the silliest and stupidest James Bond escapade to date! Uncannily, though, Sir Roger Moore's consistently *Saint*-like cool and sophisticated portrayal of the not–so–secret–and–then–space–launched British agent managed once more to out–class the outlandish script material—as did likewise composer John Barry's romantically melodic soundtrack featuring sublime singer Shirley Bassey's powerful and passionately dynamic rendition of the score's lyrical title theme song—despite most anything from novelist Ian Fleming's original story concept being unduly dispensed with!

Mike Marshall(Colonel Scott)had already launched into outer space long before, portraying Lt White in *The Phantom Planet(1961)*.

Alfie Bass(the Venice Coffin Spotter)played alongside a striking 27–year–old Sean Connery in *No Road Back(1957)* as Rudge and *Hell Drivers(1957)*as truck driver, Tinker.

Kim Fortune(RAF Officer), in case you missed him, likewise played an HMS Ranger Crewman in *The Spy Who Loved Me(1977)*.

Melinda Maxwell(uncredited as Drax's girl)is the daughter of Lois Maxwell of Miss Moneypenny fame.

This flick's sweetest treat is the extraordinarily exquisite French actress–and–*Story of O*'s Corinne Clery, playing the ill–fated Bond girl Corinne Dufour. Compared to Lois Chiles' supremely insipid Holly Goodhead, Corinne scorches the screen in her small scenes with Sir Roger Moore with her stunning sultriness! Chiles has whined publicly that she hated delivering to James Bond the line at the film's end—

"Take me around the world one more time"—exposing perhaps her conspicuous inexperience at having never been taken gloriously to heaven and back by an impassioned lover like James Bond. Well, one look from Corinne Clery's sumptuously sensual and receptive expression, once she settled slowly back for the close–up camera onto that boudoir bed, projected not only had she been torridly ravished before but that she'd profoundly relished it as well! She was no doubt extremely hot to trot lying down, even if she did represent one of the unsuspecting opposition, but I had plenty aspiring superspy troubles of my own to worry about!

§

Before ever marrying the wacko wicked witch of the South, Elizabeth, I saw some fabulous shows in south Florida mostly at the *Sunrise Musical Theatre for the Performing Arts*:

•*Johnny Carson*, comedian and *Tonight Show* host, 28–30 October 1977;

•*Jerry Lewis*, comedian and Muscular Dystrophy Association(MDA)Labor Day Telethon host, 4–6 November 1977;

•*Johnny Mathis*, ballad singer, 16–22 January 1978.

Friday night the 22nd of April 1977 at the luxurious *Galt Ocean Mile Hotel*, 3200 Galt Ocean Drive, Ft Lauderdale, Florida, the so–called *Continental Cabaret Circle of Stars* presented stage–film–and–TV actor, **Gene Barry**, star of the television serials *Bat Masterson(1958–1961)*, *Burke's Law(1963–1965)*and *Name of the Game(1968–1971)*.

At the 1191–seat *Parker Playhouse* in Ft Lauderdale, Florida I went to watch London–born child–star actor, **Roddy McDowall**, perform in Simon Gray's lacklustre play, *Otherwise Engaged*, directed by Ron Abbott, and opening Monday the 9th of January 1978.

It was March 1979 and I was back at *Florida Atlantic*

SEXCAPADES

*University(FAU)*in Boca Raton, Florida stagnating instead of studying but still profoundly relieved that I'd finally rid myself of the crazed Cuban–American witch, Elizabeth, disburdening myself of her at least temporarily, which would prove presently to be all too brief! We married in late June 1978 at Pompano Beach, Florida while we were shacked up together the preceding summer at a beachfront apartment in Highland Beach, Florida. During a short stint of teaching at a parochial high school in West Palm Beach, Florida starting in August 1978 she put me through the proverbial hell and in a matter of months made my life a complete and miserable shambles.

I paid her way to the *University of West("Worst")Florida(UWF)*back in my backwater hometown of Pensacola, Florida where she actually invited me to join her living in the marital dormitories while she finished earning her double–major bachelor's degree. In the meantime I simply subsisted that spring at FAU in Boca Raton, contemplating my irresolute and unsettled future—when that is I wasn't wasting my time and effort driving clear across the state over several weekends to Pensacola, visiting Elizabeth only to be repeatedly and spitefully expelled, typically following one of her intensely infantile and irrational outbursts, having absolutely no place to go except all the way back to south Florida.

At FAU I mis–spent most of my nights sitting in the lounge of the girl's dormitory—why?, well, that's where the girls were!—moping and mindlessly watching television. Then one fortuitous but fated night Rena had come prancing late but impressively through the dormitory lobby when she paused, stopping dead in her tracks after having caught sight of me.

§

Rena was tall, leggy, perfectly shapely and possessed of

79

a pretty, prepossessing face embraced with soft curly blond ringlets; she was remarkably reminiscent of English actress, Angela Scoular, who played Ruby Bartlett in the James Bond 007 film, *On Her Majesty's Secret Service(1969)*. She was a musical theater major and jazz pianist at the university and reveled in dancing the nights away at discotheques—and dance and move extremely provocatively she could! And when she paraded so spectacularly into any room she easily arrested all attention! The only trouble was: she was engaged to be married to an Israeli soldier—just my bad luck!

Rena had discernibly noticed and observed me sitting sulking in that dormitory lobby on numerous occasions upon returning from her regular dancing excursions. One opportune night she most graciously took it upon her most charming self to plop down into a nice cushiony chair right next to mine and proceeded then to seductively cozy up, introduce herself and get acquainted. And the rest, as they say, was history.

Once Rena awakened to my unfortunate marital troubles—and the costly emotional toll those had taken on my intensely sensitive psyche—she warmed up to me even more and resolved to devote herself to heartening me and cheering me up. On more leisurely evenings she would go along with me to a practice room in the music department building to accompany me on piano playing my trumpet. As I directly discovered she admired and idolized lyrical singer Barry Manilow and his incredible musical "modulations"— quite a quantum leap from Elizabeth's childish deification of Neil Diamond!

On one especially auspicious night Rena along with a girlfriend took me out to a nightclub contriving to tranquilize my emotional troubles by making me drunk—and I did indeed reach that point, not of no return, but of feeling no pain. Afterwards Rena dropped off her girlfriend and drove us back to the university and escorted me to my own dormitory room to bid me goodnight.

Finally we were alone together amidst the stilly quiet of the dormitory anteroom, sitting directly across from each other in chairs at the room's study carrel, gazing affectionately—almost solemnly—at one another before reaching out in the same bated breath to warmly embrace and softly kiss. Rena's lips were full, supple, responsive—expectant. Slowly I lifted up my knowing eyes to meet hers.

"I wish I had a home to take you to," I told her meaningly.

Looking suddenly smitten, she fixed her tender eyes on mine, took me warmly by my hand and led me right out of the room.

§

Rena led the way back to the dormitory lot where she parked her big car with the roomy interior; we needed its ample front–seat space to convert into a love–seat because that's where Rena's sparkling, expressive eyes communicated wordlessly she craved to be made love to.

Once she inserted into her car's 8–track player—set to *continuous* play—her tape of the seminal jazz bossa nova album, *Getz/Gilberto(1964)*, she reclined back against the driver's door, reached out and folded me in her arms to kiss and caress. I was heart–stoppingly breathless at the provocative prospect of slowly stripping off her clothes. She looked up at me, hovering over her, with a large–eyed, awestruck and even reverent wonder as I carefully unclasped her bra. I gaped in awe as her perfectly plump, pear–shaped and supple breasts fell out into my warm and waiting palms. Just as slowly and breathlessly I peeled off her scanty panties, exposing to full view the ample mound of her perfectly plump pubic shape. Finally in sight was all of her perfectly sleek, smooth and fervid flesh, faintly and softly illuminated by the dim outdoor lamplight. Gingerly she opened up her long thickset thighs, positioning herself to receive and take me in. I sprawled and slid in between her long legs, preparing to penetrate her, bracing the back of her frontward knee over the crook of my frontward forearm to spread open her legs even wider. When the hardened head of my throbbing phallus first gently touched the outermost tip of her overflowing fount I abruptly burst into her with a breathless gasp—she with a breathless outcry—plunging deeper and repeatedly into her profusely lush and gushing passage until we were both wholly overcome with the blinding delirium and euphoria of an all–consuming oblivion. Collapsing fulfilled and spent into each other's swollen bosoms we passionately embraced, kissed, caressed and coupled there in Rena's car until the break of dawn.

Rena hadn't wanted to part from me. So sometime later on she spirited me away to her upstairs dormitory room and into her springy top bed–bunk where we laid and slept more together, and where she put me out of sight beneath her bedding while her female roommate came and went in the early morning. Later on still I caught the irresistible sight of her below from behind, stripped to her panties changing tops, her curvaceous soft breasts bulging from the sides of her straight, smooth and sleek back. I couldn't help but quickly come up from behind her, clutching softly her beautifully plump and supple breasts in both of my warm palms. She let me mount her and we made love yet a third time on her dormitory room's carpeted floor.

Rarely have I regretted anything more in my entire life than parting from Rena to return to my emotionally abusive wife and Rena to her more admirable Israeli fiancé—with both of us ultimately separating from our respective partners. But never would I forget undulating the long night away with a supremely sublime young woman to the swaying jazz–and–samba–fused bossa nova rhythms and lyrical verses of Antônio Carlos Jobim, João and Astrud Gilberto(*Girl*

*From Ipanema)*and saxophonist Stan Getz. It was absolutely, altogether heavenly!

§

"A City For All Seasons," so–called, Boca Raton, Florida is populated by a sizable transplanted Northerner group of residents attributed to an influx of retiring snowbirds, so–called, flocking to south Florida from the Northeast mostly from New York City—with over 15 percent of them being Jewish. Rena had been one of them. Francine—or Fran for short—had been another.

I first spotted Fran that one sunny, warm and windy spring afternoon sitting by herself on campus at a lone picnic table area where I politely insinuated myself to chat her up. We hit it off right off, she took a shine to me, and before long we were headed together one glittering starry night to Boca Raton's small but secluded public beach where we trudgingly scaled a sloping sugary white sand dune to its crest—a solitary spot in full sight of the breezy seashore and surging surf I already knew full well and was well familiar with: because there on her favorite red blanket I'd pumped the crazed Cuban–American witch, Elizabeth, many a time over numerous nights since June 1977. Then all but two years later I was just about to romp there with Fran as well. Before we even got started making out another amorous couple had clambered up behind us, treading practically right on our heels.

"It's already occupied!" I called out irritably to them in the night; and back down they climbed.

Fran was a pretty typical college co–ed—a tall, slim, shapely, long–haired cute brunet who wore jeans and tube tops that were so delectable to peel down from the top so her perky plump breasts would pop out in the faint moonlight and right into my softly grasping hands. When it came to stripping off her scanty little panties though she skittishly uttered those infamous last feminine words.

"I've never done this before," she gasped with bated breath. "I don't know why I'm letting you do this to me."

By the way she was squirming and spreading wide open her sweet thickset thighs, nestling her plump little rump snugly into a small pocket of sand, it was most conspicuously because she had the hots for me and burned to have her brimming wet pussy pumped(and deflowered)good—supposedly for the very first time—by my dripping wet dick! And amidst the rumble of rollers breaking ashore, drowning out her outcries, she received and took in all the way the full shtuping, thumping extent of what she pantingly lusted after!

Fran had acted quite sentimental about our steamy seaside coupling and, together with my kind–hearted Chinese roommate for that term, bid me a fond goodbye and saw me off on the day of my departure once more in May 1979 for Pensacola, Florida.

By the end of August 1979 after a transfer of required course credit from *Florida Atlantic University(FAU)*, the *University of West(Worst)Florida*, in turn, conferred on me its second worthless bachelor of arts(BA)degree in economics.

§

The crazed Cuban–American witch, Elizabeth, had resumed making my life a complete and miserable shambles so nothing had changed until I was sick of the situation and finally fed up enough to act...to *shift the scene!*

Days before Christmas 1979 Elizabeth had moved with my help from the marital dormitory to a private dormitory room across the *University of West(Worst)Florida(UWF)*campus before heading home to visit her parents in Key West, Florida. I prepared to travel in January 1980 to Tampa,

Florida to transfer temporarily to the *University of South Florida(USF)*simply to escape the shrew. For a precious few days before my appointed departure date I stayed in her dormitory room with an incredibly angelic young 24–year–old Chinese girl from Taiwan whose acquaintance I'd only just recently made but who in time would become my second wife. In the meantime I was bent upon getting my own back and going out with a big *bang*—or *two!*

Maid Marian was a mightily busty(even in her thick sweater top), lusty and slutty looking brunet whom at a study table in the university library I'd met and picked up, inviting her to the student rathskeller for some refreshment before being invited in turn to her dormitory room where before long in her hot little bed I proceeded to bonk her throughout the night. Poetically just enough, Marian's upstairs bedroom window was in full view of the marital dormitory bedroom below—the sight at which I gazed with sheer delight!—in the adjacent building where the crazed Cuban–American witch, Elizabeth, had resumed making my life a complete miserable shambles over roughly the past half–year!

Then there was Twila, a cute, chubby but buxom blond who worked in the circulation–and–subscription department at a local community weekly newspaper I'd for years written for, and who'd long since lusted to get into my pants, as she most lewdly put it. Following a drunken Christmas holiday party she invited me to—thrown Saturday night the 22nd of December 1979 at the recreation hall at *Royal Arms* apartments at 5655 North 9th Avenue—I finally accommodated her in her parked car, necking heatedly and feeling up her curvaceous titties beneath her disheveled bra, she groping and stroking my dripping dick through my wet pants.

Then there came into my head yet another ingenious but still poetically just inspiration: I directed Twila to drive us to the university martial dormitories on UWF campus and stealthily insinuate ourselves with my kept key into the very same vacated apartment where I'd lived since June 1979 with the crazed Cuban–American witch, Elizabeth, but which by then was conspicuously occupied by a fresh married couple presumably away on vacation for the holiday. At least that's what I'd banked on when I'd most rashly put both of our hot and horny asses on the line by getting some of Twila's randy ass in that very same darkened bed where I'd laid Elizabeth all that time before. We lucked out by hastily getting off and then getting well out of it without incident—and without getting caught trespassing(and wildly romping)upon another couple's rented bed, which we left decidedly disheveled, which in turn must've left the returning couple decidedly confounded once they got back! Even in my decidedly drunken condition slutty Twila had deemed it a "good lay" so it'd been well worth the trip! "You'll *always* be my friend," she wrote me on 4 February 1980, "no matter what you do or where you go in life."

Friday night the 28th of December 1979 at *Cordova Mall* cinema at 5100 North 9th Avenue Twila invited me to see *Star Trek: The Motion Picture(1979)*—the first flick in the long–running major motion picture film franchise based on the original classic *Star Trek(1966–1969)*television series, cancelled a decade earlier.

After the flick Twila drove us roughly 25 miles east of Pensacola to Navarre Beach, Florida, part of the barrier Santa Rosa Island on the Gulf of Mexico, where much of the film sequel, *Jaws 2(1978)*, was filmed. Hotel scenes in the flick were filmed at the *Navarre Beach Holiday Inn*, a complex subsequently destroyed by Hurricane Ivan in September 2004—and not far from which we bonked on the beach before the night was out!

Sunday night the 23rd of December 1979 I somehow got invited to a private party on UWF campus in Dorm 68, where I met a tall, voluptuous, top–heavy brunet co–ed with a full mouth whose long dark hair reached to the small of her back. Her name was Barbara and she was just 21 or so—four years younger than myself.

We wound up in her own private dorm room, enfolded and fondling on the floor next to her bed rather than on it though we once came very close to being in it together. We were warmly making out in softly flickering candlelight to some mellow music she was playing on her stereo turntable.

My roaming right hand slid lightly across her inner thick-set thighs, gently petting her ample pubic mound, mildly massaging her sweet crotch at the creases of her jeans with my exploring fingertips; surely she was gushing underneath.

"IfyoukeeptouchingmelikethatIwon'tbeabletotakeitmuch longer,"shefinallyraspedbreathlessly,ripeandreadytobetaken.

Stupidly—out of some irresolute scruples—I stopped and Barbara became one bodacious chick who got away!

Presently this aspiring superspy would be making a rather compulsory trip once more to south Florida before making a rather remarkable comeback!

§

By March 1980 this aspiring superspy was back with a vengeance at the *University of West(Worst)Florida(UWF)*in Pensacola, Florida and on the offensive, attending classes full–time while working regular part–time(the retail euphemism for just under regular full–time)four miles distant from the university campus at a mall bookstore to which I either biked, hiked, hitch–hiked or in due time borrowed the cars of caring and concerned friends to drive myself to work when they weren't driving me themselves. Living alone in my own private dormitory room I was still screwing regularly my crazed Cuban–American witch of a wife, who was still living across campus in her own private dormitory room before finally sending herself packing back to mama and papa in June 1980 to Key West, Florida. In the meantime I was also screwing regularly my latest love interest, a perfectly innocent and virtuous little Chinese girl of 24 from Taiwan who ably and secretly aided my return from Tampa, Florida every step of the way since I escaped temporarily the previous January. But they wouldn't be the only two females I'd be making it with by any means. Over the next several months until the year's end I'd be running myself and my over–revved libido ragged by indiscriminately and promiscuously screwing every easy, consenting and willing wet pussy in sight!

§

In 1980 they showed up at either the bookstore or on the university campus but either way they came brimming!

Right off the bat on Tuesday the 15th of April 1980 a somewhat scruffy but cute hands–in–her–pockets brunet teenager of 18 or so named Jackie took a quick shine to me and became my first mall groupie, letting me drive her straight to my dormitory room on campus right after my workshift to doff her dungarees and do her before taking her out to eat chicken(at *Jerry's Drive–In*)and then driving her in the neighborhood of *Washington High School* at 6000 College Parkway to her parental home at 1601 Bakalane Avenue, which was roughly in the university vicinity; she dropped around the bookstore next three nights later on the 18th to meet up with me after work. She'd be back to hang around a lot with me in times to come.

Tuesday the 13th of May 1980 I treated Jackie to fast food during my mall bookstore workshift.

Jackie wouldn't drop by the bookstore again until Saturday the 9th of August 1980 when she invited me out to a nearby saloon called *Chan's* to drink a couple of London bass ales together—after which we found our way biking round midnight to a secluded spot located north of the mall off a woodsy footpath where I spread my shirt on the grassy ground for her to lie down so I could do her again, escorting her home afterwards, stopping for a lemon–lime *Sprite* soda at the nearby *Waffle House* chain restaurant on our way.

Jackie picked me up two nights later on Monday the 11th at the mall and I escorted her to her house on Bakalane Avenue, stopping for a *Coke* at the *Whataburger* fast food chain restaurant on our way, screwing her on the ground right beneath her own bedroom window but creaming rather prematurely out of anxiety at the unaccustomed situation.

Five nights later on Saturday the 16th we had drinks after the mall closed at *Chan's* again and then biked the four miles to my campus dormitory room where we fucked, cuddled and caressed for roughly an hour until well past midnight before she had to leave to return home; on Tuesday the 19th she dropped in the bookstore in the late afternoon, hugging me and nuzzling her head into my chest.

Six nights later on Friday night the 22nd of August 1980 we met for a movie at the mall—the Peter Sellers comedy film, *The Fiendish Plot of Fu Manchu(1980)*—heading afterwards one block shy of the main university campus entrance for the *Nativity of Our Lord Catholic Church* at 9945 Hillview Drive where we securely chained our bikes to a metal lamp–post. Then into the woods again we went near University Parkway to quite sacrilegiously but unceremoniously screw to our genitalia's content!

That night Jackie was lying supine in a downward sloping, head–rushing position while I was pumping her.

Lately she'd been growing much more affectionate and cuddly with me.

"What do you crave more," I rather stupidly asked her amidst our gasping pants, "affection or passion?"

"I have no answer to that!" she rather astutely answered.

Clever girl!

Afterwards we biked together to the *Lil' General* convenience store where I treated us to two *Heath* English–style toffee ice cream bars and especially for her a cheeseburger sandwich and a *Nehi* grape–flavored soda.

Despite our nearly ten–year age difference we paled around together like a couple of kids into early 1982.

Friday night the 29th of August 1980 after the mall closed at the *Space Port* game room Jackie beat me badly at a game she introduced me to called *Skyhawk*—though once I got the hang of it I presently played doubles against two other youthful challengers scoring in excess of 27,000!

My favorite video arcade game became *Atari Inc's Asteroids*(just released in 1979)—at which time my earliest high score exceeded just 11,000. In times to come I greatly improved: Friday the 12th of September 1980 my score exceeded 14,000; Saturday the 27th of September 1980 it exceeded 15,000. Sunday the 18th of January 1981 I hit 18,290. Saturday the 24th of January 1981 I hit 22,660; a little better Friday the 27th of February 1981, hitting 22,881. Out of practice for awhile my scoring rather regressed in months to come. Saturday the 15th of August 1981 I hit 16,190. Friday the 4th of September 1981 I hit 19,080. By Wednesday the 9th of September I made a marked comeback, scoring in excess of 28,000! Tuesday the 15th of September my score exceeded 32,000!—regressing slightly Friday the 25th of September to around 26,000 and Saturday the 3rd of October to around 31,000. Tuesday the 29th of December 1981 I regressed again to around 21,000—even more to around 15,000 on Thursday the 31st. Saturday the 9th of January 1982 I hit around 25,000, regressing again to around 21,000 Thursday the 14th. Friday the 5th of February 1982 I hit around 25,000 again.

Months later at the so–called *Sweet Shop* in Tallahassee, Florida on Tuesday the 14th of September 1982 I hit a high score of 35,620! Back at the *Sweet Shop* a week later on Tuesday the 21st I regressed but still scored a 29,200–plus

"WIN." Tuesday the 16th of November 1982 at the *Sweet Shop* I hit another high score in excess of 37,000! And again Wednesday the 30th of March 1983, scoring in excess of 38,200, but regressing again to 20,000–plus by the 1st of April! Wednesday the 25th of July 1984 I scored 16,309 after not playing for over roughly one year.

§

Friday the 18th of April 1980 an exceptionally pretty and comely young chick named Tama(nicknamed "TI" for short) waltzed into the bookstore to chat me up; she was impressed by the interest I expressed in her various pursuits—amongst which she aspired to become a county deputy sheriff. As it turned out she worked as a one–woman security task force for the nearby *Sears* mid–range chain department store; she stopped by the bookstore to greet me once more Wednesday the 30th of April 1980.

Monday the 5th of May 1980 Tama stopped by the bookstore to greet me, strolling along with me around the mall after my workshift, treated me to a *Coke* at *Chick–fil–A*, the second–largest chicken–based fast–food chain in America specializing in chicken entrées headquartered in College Park, Georgia; she paused to make a wishing well–wish! Afterwards she showed me her security office at *Sears*, where she led me to the store's "rec hall"—by way of a trip on the store's freight elevator—to buy me another vending machine *Coke* before I left.

Later on that night Tama telephoned me at my private dorm room on UWF campus, inviting me over to her place, a snug and small mobile home where she lived in a nearby neighborhood with her daughterly child, who happened to be asleep when I drove over. She told me an incredibly disheartening story about her husband abandoning her to run off with some 15–year–old adolescent girl!

Before long our couch–bound chitchat while drinking
Pepsi cola upgraded(or downgraded depending upon your
point of view)to drinking vodka–and–orange juice screw-
drivers and grappling with one another on her carpeted living room floor to her rather empty and unresistant protests.

"It's not right!" she asserted. "I'm not good at it!"

Yes, well, she most assuredly had her bedside contracep-
tive foam near at hand and within ready reach! In her big
rearward bed her incredibly baby–soft, supple and cuddly
body had me writhing with excitement; her blush–colored
skin was incredibly fleshy and grab–able!

Coupled deep with her I undulated languidly atop her
in a pelvis–down–in–brush–across–her–breasts–with–my–
chest–up–and–down–and–in–again maneuver which I'd
long since discovered turned girls on and really got them
going!

"You're *good!*" she emphatically declared.

"Leave when you're through," she said at first, decisively
changing her mind afterward.

Watching the Tuesday sunrise through a little window
alongside Tama was incredibly serene, tranquil and warm
though she arose early during the weekday morning children's television series, *Captain Kangaroo(1955–1984)*, making us and her baby daughter a breakfast with orange juice
and then making ready to leave and attend a morning junior
college class. She was inexpressibly pretty in nothing but her
scanty panties as she dressed in–between affectionate and
tender kisses to my lips.

"Don't tell anyone my rates," she jested playfully in parting.

Just two nights later Thursday the 8th Tama invited me
back over to her place but that time played a taunting game
of hard–to–get. Three times I hopped a fence, getting into
the car to leave, and three times she summoned me back
until she finally demanded, "Come back you son–of–a–bitch

and take me to bed!"

I did and again she was incredibly delectable! The morning after on the 9th she brought me piping–hot cocoa to bed.

During my workshift that Friday at the mall bookstore Tama stopped by with a tall and pretty girl in tow to give me a pickle to eat; Saturday on the 10th I visited her at her *Sears* security office and she took me once more to the "rec hall" to introduce me to a couple lady operators she'd mentioned me to.

At other times she brought me from the store popcorn or my favorite store candy: chocolate nonpareil wafers or malted milk balls. Sunday night on the 11th we were back together after I rode a bike over to her place making love again. Following breakfast the next morning she drove me and my bike back to the university campus, came along to my private dormitory room, making inconspicuous love with me beneath my blanket while her baby daughter obliviously watched television! After my mall bookstore workshift that Monday the 12th Tama brought me popcorn from *Sears*, packed my bike in her car and drove me back to my campus dorm room; I biked her little girl to their car parked behind the department store—where we met up the next afternoon during our workshifts to visit her security office, the store "rec hall," and stroll the mall together, licking ice cream cones and stealing sweet smooches.

Wednesday the 14th of May 1980 Tama drove along with her baby daughter to pick me up at the university campus and take me to her place to make love again, making me breakfast and bringing me back to campus the next morning. Early that Thursday the 15th I drove to her place to sleep happily alongside her for a couple of hours before she had to depart for the day.

So it went until *Memorial Day* Monday the 26th came around but instead of watching the *Indianapolis 500* we were making love again. And though she was fond of then relatively unknown Dan Fogelberg, Tama let me study for an upcoming test lying perched atop her bed listening to WMEZ(EAZY)94 FM, making me breakfast before driving me—and my bike—back to campus the next morning.

"I'm glad you're not working as a street cop," Tama cracked once she picked me up on UWF campus Tuesday the 3rd of June 1980 after a night class, "you'd run right past the surveillance."

She'd parked her car behind a tree and I'd dashed toward another car flashing its lights in the lot where she'd told me she'd be waiting. Turning about I spotted her instantly and got into her car.

"I didn't think you'd be playing games with your car–parking," I said wearily, "and would be where you said you'd be."

Saturday the 7th of June 1980 Tama invited me over for a sit–down dinner with her parents and brother at their home at 276 St Augustine Drive.

Then in a rather drastic and inexplicable turnabout on what I'd normally consider to be a most fortuitous Friday the 13th, Tama wigged out—weirding me out!—as if she were on the rag and ordered me to "get out" of her store security office once I stopped by briefly to visit.

"I don't need your friendship," she said adamantly.

"You'd better watch your expressions!" she admonished me further about my doubtless dumbfounded demeanor.

"You'd better watch your over–reactions," I cooly told her before leaving, writing her off as some whacked out psycho–neurotic chick, and never looked back.

Thursday the 24th of July 1980 she passed by outside the bookstore in the mall cheerfully *waving* at me! Go figure!

§

Sunday the 1st of June 1980 I chatted up and picked up

outside the theatre building on UWF campus a hot little number—a little older—wearing scanty gym shorts named Doreen who before the day was through had invited me over to her place to visit and stay over, spending a most innocent night together: she actually slept on the living room sofa, letting me sleep in her bed.

Doreen was merely a lodger renting a room in the rather huge house at 3422 McLean Avenue of a young but more womanly divorcé and daycare worker with two kids named Penny who aspired to be a nurse, and who outspokenly wondered what had drawn me to Doreen whom she'd always thought was "too hyper." And I had to outspokenly admit and own up that it had been her alluring legs! Though I was awakened earlier Monday the next morning by chirping and window–pecking birds it was Penny, and not Doreen, who let me sleep in late before letting me shower in her bath, heated me toast for breakfast and drove me herself back to the university campus.

It wouldn't be until Saturday the 4th of October 1980 though when Penny would invite me over one night to visit her at home where she happened to be alone and on her own but upset over some "emotional problems" her first–grade son was experiencing.

On her couch we cuddled and chatted until well past midnight.

"I feel like a little girl in your arms," she said.

After a couple of hours she invited me to rest in her bedroom. I hadn't been rushing things but by then I knew for sure that she longed to be treated more like a woman than a girl, little or otherwise!

Once we were reclined together on her bed we undertook the natural progression of closely cuddling, softly caressing and tenderly kissing. My warm palms explored the fervid flesh of her body through her flimsy nightgown, beneath her bra, across the silken smoothness of her stomach, down and up again along the supple softness of her thickset thighs, kissing more deeply and deliriously until she was squirming tortuously beneath me.

Abruptly she expressed apprehension at having recently inserted into herself an intrauterine device(IUD)and at being midway into her monthly menstrual cycle.

"This is crazy!" she repeated at least twice. More infamous last feminine words!

By that time I'd already stripped us both and we were beyond that point of no return.

I was kissing her softly all over from head to toe, tongueing her tenderly between her legs to wet and melt her because she had tightened at first.

"Such sweet kisses," she murmured.

"I want to love you badly," I whispered to her, sliding atop her and in–between her legs. "You *do* want me, don't you?"

She nodded mutely.

"Open your legs more...wider," I gently prodded her, panting slightly. "Let me in you...Take me in you...gently..."

Penny was no longer concerned with gentleness and began tugging hard at my hips, heaving upwards against me.

"Do you want me now...all of me?"

She nodded even more discernibly.

So I gave it to her—all of it.

"My God, you pressed all the right buttons," she complimented me afterwards. "You're a good lover. You've had lots of practice, huh?"

"Was it *really* good for you?" I'd ask that cornball question for the first and last time ever.

"You don't have to ask that," she said assuredly. "You *know* it was!"

"You just like seducing younger men," I kidded her.

"Yes—to boost my ego," she quipped but just half in jest, I thought.

"Now what am I going to do with you?" she pondered

aloud.

"Invite me back," I countered coolly, smiling.

Though I hadn't realized it at the time—some six years before actually relocating to the western coastal state—I'd just fucked my first California chick for Penny was actually from Santa Barbara.

Penny telephoned me the next day to confess that she felt both awkward and confused about our tryst the night before, suggesting that sex was supposed to be at once sacred and carefree, but expressing sweetly her appreciation for the "sensitivity" of my lovemaking.

Four days later on Wednesday the 8th of October Penny drove me together with her little daughter to an eatery called *Gino's* for soda.

Saturday night the 11th of October I visited Penny once more at her house, helping her complete a college financial aid form; we necked on her couch but she wouldn't fuck.

By mid–June 1980 I was awarded my Associate of Science(AS)degree in law enforcement by the junior college which recorded my completion of its graduation require-ments ass–backwards at the end of July 1980.

§

Late Monday night the 28th of July 1980 I took some chick back to my private dorm room whom I can't really recall named Susan.

She snuggled with me in my bed and stayed overnight until early the next morning, necking and fondling but not fucking per "our agreement" of restraint since she had no birth control pills.

"Lover," she kept on calling me. "You drive me crazy. You feel so nice."

I kissed her all over her naked body.

She directly left on her own after daybreak but declined my offers to walk her to her car in my robe or direct her off campus.

§

Tuesday the 23rd of September 1980 I met a cute dynamic roommate duo named Kat and Leta at some "submarine social" on the university campus. And two nights later on the 25th—truer to the more promiscuous spirit of her own nickname—Kat would be chitchatting with me in my private dormitory room, reclining on my twin bed until I'd finally dim my nightstand lamp, neck with her, doff her tight–fitting jeans and fuck her before she ever knew what had hit her—hurriedly at first, more leisurely a second time a little later on.

"This only happens in the movies," she gasped breathlessly, claiming that it didn't "normally" happen.

More infamous last feminine words.

"You're here," I assured her. "It happened. So welcome to the real world!"

Early the next morning on the 26th I loaned Kat my robe so that she could dress and, confirming that the way out was clear, discreetly depart.

"How chivalrous," she exclaimed. "What a gentleman!"

"Oh," Kat said once I hugged her snugly in passing later on that night at a campus fraternity party, "you can do that anytime."

And that very night Kat returned the favor by loaning me out temporarily to her friend Leta after inviting me over to slumber with candlelight on Leta's big "comforter" bed, making herself suddenly scarce and leaving me alone with Leta, who let me neck and cop feels with her but who wouldn't fuck.

"I know what I'm doing," Leta said, insisting sternly on stroking my genitals instead.

And I supposed she did know so I readily agreed.

§

At one of those drunken on–campus university keg parties Thursday night the 16th of October 1980 I met a tallish, pale but shapely and thickset young lady of 29 named Jenny who had short but straight–waved raven–black hair. From first stuffing her into the cramped chest of an ice–making machine("I don't believe you did that!" she exclaimed)to later necking outside on a wooden bench I finally found my way into that over–concealing blouse of hers and discovered she was possessed of wonderfully full–fleshed breasts. So right off I was hooked even if she wasn't possessed of the most attractive features. My God, what a body this chick had!

"I must fight temptation," she said, apologizing for having to rise early the next morning for an employment interview, so I saw her off to her private dormitory room.

By the time I'd already been fucking regularly a racy young chick on campus named Mary Jo toward the end of October, Jenny showed up at the university rathskeller hoping I'd be there, she'd admit later on.

After first escorting back to her room a big beautiful black girl named Dalles, who was likewise part and parcel of that university rathskeller crowd, I made my way across campus Thursday night the 23rd of October 1980 to visit at her invitation Jenny, who'd already slipped into her flimsy nightie and was waiting expectantly to let me in to promptly screw her!

She told me she'd been "discriminating," since she hadn't had a man in her bed for an entire year, saying as well that screwing me had been "well worth the wait."

Talk about being at the right place at the right time!

Afterward I stayed with her for awhile but presently excused myself, albeit apologetically, tucking her snugly into bed, taking her room keys, going out and locking her in securely before sliding her room keys back inside beneath her door—a recurring practice I'd cultivated for departing late from the rooms of college co–ed chicks I'd be screwing all over campus right and left!

On the night of the university campus *Oktoberfest* celebration I was jumping that sprightly chick named Mary Jo at her private dormitory room. Round midnight Sunday the 26th of October 1980 after *Oktoberfest* I was jumping Jenny at hers. After drinking together only one glass of wine Jenny would exclaim that our fucking had felt incredibly "good and wonderful."

"Oh, that's nice," Jenny said once I greeted her with a cheek kiss in passing on campus Tuesday the 28th.

Late–night on the eve of All Hallow's Eve I found the word "Death" ominously painted in red on my private dormitory room door. But late on Halloween night itself I was quite alive and kicking—or rather fucking Jenny in her private dormitory room quite lively!—first plowing into her upright against the wall and then, playing grab–ass, plunking her gently down, fucking her forcefully on her carpet!

Sleeping with Jenny until late the next morning I came alive again only to find her eyes riveted, gazing intently at me.

Thursday the 6th of November 1980 I found a note from Jenny at my private dormitory room saying she needed me *"tonight!"*

When I arrived at Jenny's private dormitory room I found her gone but a note from her stuck to her door telling me it was open—and another unfinished note to me placed on her bed.

Presently Jenny returned with a friend named Janet who, climbing the dormitory building steps, promptly scolded me, flipping the finger, "You'd *better* be up there, boy!"

So what was all the urgent to–do about?

Well, Jenny of all things happened to be turning 30 and was in a complete panic about it and so she had a pressing need to be fucked. So naturally I promptly obliged her.

"I love having you in me," she repeated frequently. "It's so good. You can warm my bed anytime. Before I loved being in my bed alone. Now I love having you in it."

§

At some drunken on–campus university fraternity party I caught up with a cute, slender but shapely, spirited, short blond–haired chick named Mary Jo, turning just 28 at the first of the upcoming month of November, who'd swiveled her pelvis to music very provocatively the night before at the keg party where I'd just encountered Jenny so up close and personal. Friday night the 17th of October 1980 though Jenny wasn't about but Mary Jo was and she presently invited me to her private dormitory room where we heatedly necked, stripped and listened to music, but she wouldn't fuck because she was going through her monthly menstrual cycle—as if I gave a flying fuck about that!—though she exclaimed that I'd made her come by stroking her tight gushing pussy with my forefingers!

"Suck me," she moaned once I worked my exploring mouth into her T–shirt. "I *want* you! I *want* you to make love to me!"

So once I even wormed my over–anxious dick into her scanty panties and into her resistant wet pussy but came prematurely.

"I'm so cruel," she reassured me apologetically. "You really turn me on...You're so nice...I like you a lot...You're so cuddly...After you've had more rest maybe we can take up where we left off...!"

And would we indeed!

Mary Jo invited me afresh into her private dormitory room the very next Saturday night the 18th. And she was one chick who liked to be fucked good and hard and wasn't embarrassed or ashamed to shout it out aloud!

"Yeah! Oh yeah! Fuck me! C'mon! Come to me!" she

screamed when I slammed her!

So that night I pumped her good and hard—*twice!*—plunging her so deeply she affirmed how "far" I'd penetrated her.

Whatever, I rated two separate sweet servings of English muffins, jelly and milk throughout the time afterward—some six hours or so more—we spent cuddling and sleeping together between dawn and noon.

"You're so nice and cuddly to have around," she told me heartily.

Just two nights later on Monday the 20th I was fucking Mary Jo in my own private dormitory room when she kindly complimented me, "You're tender and know how to treat a woman."

And the very next day after that she was loaning out to me her rather battered white green–roofed *Dodge Dart* compact car to drive myself to work, run errands and sometimes go off on some recreational excursions.

After the very first time I borrowed her car on Tuesday the 21st I returned to express my appreciation by promptly attacking and fucking Mary Jo in her private dormitory room at midday—a *nooner!*

"Right in the afternoon," she exclaimed. "*That* was nice!"

Love in the afternoon indeed!

Twice more we were getting it on vigorously later on that very night; I stayed and slept overnight and she saw me off early the next morning with a disposable cup of sweetened hot tea.

By the next day Mary Jo was sweetly keeping a photograph of me propped up at her desk.

"I like looking at it while I study," she said.

Friday night the 24th of October 1980 following the campus *Oktoberfest* revelry I headed straight with Mary Jo for her private dormitory room where we did some spry celebrating of our own spiritedly thumping the night away!

SEXCAPADES

Tuesday the 28th of October 1980 following a night work–shift at the mall—to which she'd given me a gray sweater to wear—I was back over at her place late at night fucking her again because she affirmed she'd been feeling powerfully horny!

"Fuck me! Fuck me!" she commanded, screaming. "You're so *good!*"

Afterward she calmed herself quietly down.

"I like the way you touch me," she muttered affectionately. "You're so gentle and tender."

Then she expressed her preference to sleep with me and pretend to be "domestic."

It was tragic to think in retrospect that 13 extremely unlucky people were killed roughly a month earlier in the worst calamitous terrorist attack in Germany's history when a deadly pipe bomb loaded with 1.39 kilograms of TNT and mortar shells exploded inside a trash can at the main entrance showers of the actual *Oktoberfest* at the Theresienwiese meadow at Munich in Bavaria!

Tuesday night the 11th of November 1980 I engaged with Mary Jo in not so much a sympathy as a sympa*thetic* fuck when I found her drunk in her private dormitory room grieving mournfully over the passing away of her step–father; I felt supremely sorry for her.

"Your poem was beautiful—your note was beautiful— you are beautiful," Mary Jo once wrote me in a note after asking me to write her a poem about unrequited love, "…I love the child in you—don't ever lose it…I just wanted to say hello and thank you for being my friend."

§

About the very same time I'd met Jenny I also met Dalles, a big, beautiful black girl with large eyes, perfectly smooth and soft cheeks, and utterly luscious lips.

Thursday night the 23rd of October 1980 right after I'd jumped Jenny for the very first late–night time at her private dormitory room—after I'd first escorted Dalles from the university campus rathskeller back to her private dormitory room—I returned very early that very same morning to...*do* Dalles! And to the soulful sounds of Teddy Pendergrass no less *do* her I did!

Dalles kindly complimented me, "You're so fine and passionate."

Quite curiously, I thought, she voluntarily assured me that she'd divulge our copulation to no one, assuring me as well that I was "welcome to come over anytime without being under any obligation."

After tucking Dalles back into bed, I took her room keys, went out, locked her in securely, sliding her keys back beneath her door. And then I headed back for my own private dormitory room, sleeping extremely tired and spent throughout late the next afternoon.

Tuesday the 4th of November 1980 I was back doing Dalles in her private dormitory room where she served me a bologna and ham sandwich with milk—this time to the romantic melodies of Johnny Mathis!

"It's *so* good!" she repeated frequently.

She invited me to accompany her home to Miramar, Florida in Broward County for Christmas but I wasn't able to go along.

"I missed you," she told me late Thursday night the 20th of November 1980 when we were making it again in her private dormitory room amidst relishing chocolate chip cookies, milk and, yes, Johnny Mathis melodies—four nights after I'd happily happened upon a lovely, tall, buxom and curvaceous lady named Cindy!

"It's so good," Dalles told me rapturously overnight Monday the 1st of December 1980 after we ate spaghetti together at her private dorm room. "You're like something

I'd like to wrap up, take home and save for a rainy day." Someone else besides my Chinese girlfriend needed to "spoil" me, she said.

Well, the Christmas gift–giving season was indeed on the horizon!

§

Saturday the 1st of November 1980 at a post–Halloween costume party I made the acquaintance of a comely young girl named Karen, who after a late–night breakfast invited me driving to follow her in her car as she guided me to her apartment, located on Scenic Highway, where she hurried- ly made her bed whilst I made use of her bathroom. By the time she used her bathroom I'd already stripped off my clothes, turned out the lights and gotten into her bed and be- neath her bedding. Still clothed she came over to sit beside me on the bed. Gently I drew her to me and undressed her slowly underneath her covers.

This girl was really gorgeous, fleshy, full, exception- ally supple but supremely firm, especially her bosom—and a dead ringer for actress *Jill St John(Tiffany Case in 1971's Diamonds Are Forever)!* But once she was naked and fucking she unexpectedly acted curiously reluctant about the entire encounter.

"You come on strong," she told me, teary–eyed, right in the thick of dipping the wick, "but you're doing a good job of it!"

Fidgety, she was anxious to tell me some unspecified thing, fretted about her landlady, felt uncomfortable about taking home to bed someone strange, stressing that I couldn't stay overnight. Then she suddenly maundered about being a mean woman who cussed and smoked but thought that love was important.

To each their own but presently I politely excused myself,

dressed and left. To me she sounded like she was scrupulously screwing around on somebody who might be pretty upset about it—and who I wouldn't want to run into accidentally!

§

Sunday night the 16th of November 1980 I casually encountered a tall, full–figured and well–formed young woman with long, raven black hair named Cindy playing the lone piano late in the lodge–like university Commons building, asking her if I could accompany her on my flugelhorn and we wound up playing along together until past midnight.

Right off we hit it off and before long we were wandering around together on the raftered second–floor landings, going back and forth restlessly between opposite wings beneath the timber crossbeams where we were heatedly making out in the empty upstairs lounges and sitting rooms. Finally we found our way into a darkened classroom in a far corner corridor.

"Why are you so damned irresistible?" Cindy gasped as I doffed her dungarees and laid her down onto the carpet.

"This is dangerous," I said, plunging her on the floor.

"Exciting though," she said, breathless.

It was nearly dawn when I finally walked her to her dormitory room, telling her I wanted to see her again, even though she disbelieved that I'd been dying to kiss her and thought she was a very lovely lady!

Cindy soon began believing in me more when I was over early the very next Monday morning the 17th, making love with her until nearly noon in her dormitory room while her roommate happened happily to be away. She was the first girl for a long time whom I confided in about the rather grueling life I'd been leading over the past four years or so. She had a warm Goldie Hawn–style smile, a warm–hearted nature and a compassionate understanding of my predicament. And before long I began feeling the powerfully familiar and recognizable pangs of falling gradually but irrevocably in love with her.

"I love what you do to me—just everything," she told me feelingly late Saturday night the 22nd of November 1980 when we were intimately familiar again, making love twice to *Cat Stevens* music. She appreciated it as a compliment when I told her she'd been the first woman I'd met since April whom I wanted to spend any extended length of time with.

Tuesday night the 25th we'd time for only a rather forceful quickie in her dormitory while her roommate was gone dining. Before the year was out we got it on several more times, whether at my private dormitory room or on the floor of her not–so–private dormitory room to quiet the shtup–thumping.

Thanksgiving Thursday the 27th of November 1980 Cindy invited me to accompany her to Chipley, county seat of Washington County in northwest Florida, to ride horses at the small farm of friends of her family, who lived in Lynn Haven in Bay County, north of Panama City, Florida.

Of my crazed Cuban–American witch of a wife Cindy once sweetly said Saturday the 29th of November 1980: "I think *she* gave up a lot."

Somehow or other it was quickly becoming an exceptionally complicated Christmastime season at year's end 1980!

FIVE: *FOR YOUR AYES ONLY*

"Last night was absolutely wonderful. For some reason, being with you makes me very happy. It's not only the sex, it's talking, touching and holding...It's feeling that you care and knowing that I care—although I'm not sure why."—**Jenny, 7 February 1981, following a double whammy!**

For Your Eyes Only*(1981)*, starring Sir Roger Moore once more as not–so–secret British agent James Bond 007, and marking a return of sorts to Bond's grittier, tougher and more serious and realistic roots—more in keeping with and faithful to the original novel source material—is my all–time favorite of what is arguably Sir Roger Moore's strongest and best appearance as Bond. Even at age 53 his performance isn't so much nonchalantly *Saint*–like as it is sheer *crispy* cool and a joy to watch! Bravo, Sir Roger! It was even an exceedingly re-freshing change as well to see Bond cavorting with a wom-anly character in the fine and comely form of Countess Lisl von Schlaf, played perfectly by Australian actress Cassandra Harris, who at 33 was actually in a more carnally credible age range for being a so–called "Bond girl." And despite Sir Roger Moore proclaiming *his* Bond wouldn't commit such a cold–blooded act, it was indeed entirely consistent with Ian Fleming's James Bond to give assassin Emile Locque's pre-cariously cliff–perched car the nudge needed by deliberately kicking it to send it hurtling down the deadly escarpment. As the *real* James Bond put it in the *real* "Living Daylights" short story:

"Look, my friend," said Bond wearily, "I've got to commit a murder tonight. Not you. Me. So be a good chap and *stuff* it, would you?"

Take diligent note as there Bond could very well be ad-dressing any number of his latter–day, supposedly "progres-sive," politically correct, revisionist critics. So let's cut out all the bull–crap, shall we? Bond may not like it at times, but he's an extremely efficient, calculating and meticulous crown–paid killer—and he knows it full well. Period.

Controversial or not, finally, that shot showcasing the sleek model wearing thong–like shorts holding a crossbow and framing Bond between her lithe legs is one of the fran-chise's hottest teaser artwork posters ever!

Julian Glover(Aristotle Kristatos)made impressive appearances in classical horror flicks like *Theatre of Death(1966)* as Charles Marquis and *Hammer Horror's Quatermass and the Pit(1967)*as the stubbornly skeptical Colonel Breen.

Jill Bennett(Jacoba Brink)most notably played Peter Cushing's wife, Jane Maitland, in horror writer Robert Bloch's, *The Skull(1965)*, for *Amicus* horror productions.

Michael Gothard(Emile Leopold Locque)likewise had already appeared most notably as Keith in the horror flick, *Scream and Scream Again(1970)*.

James Villiers(Bill Tanner)as well played Corbeck in *Hammer Horror's Blood From The Mummy's Tomb(1971)*and George in *Amicus'* horror anthology, *Asylum(1972)*.

John Wells(Denis Thatcher)had earlier played Q's Assistant in *Casino Royale(1967)*.

In addition to playing Smithers twice in both *Eyes Only* and *Octopussy(1983)*, uncredited the first time, Jeremy Bulloch had already appeared as an HMS Ranger Crewman in *The Spy Who Loved Me(1977)*.

Lenny Rabin(ski–jump spectator)played serial uncredited bit parts in *Goldfinger(1964)*as an American gangster, *On Her Majesty's Secret Service(1969)*as a casino guest, *The Spy Who Loved Me(1977)*as a Liparus Crewman and *Octopussy(1983)* as a bidder at Sotheby's.

Robert Rietty(Ernst Stavro Blofeld's voice)did the uncredited voices as well for John Strangways in *Dr. No(1962)*, Emilio Largo in *Thunderball(1965)*and Tiger Tanaka in *You Only Live Twice(1967)*, and played both the Casino Baccarat Official in *On Her Majesty's Secret Service(1969)*and the Italian Minister in Sean Connery's overlong–delayed return as 007 in *Never Say Never Again(1983)*, dubbing as well Marcel Steiner/Dallas Adams in the frightening *Amicus* horror anthology, *From Beyond The Grave(1973)*.

Lizzie Warville(pool babe)played a Russian girl earlier in *Moonraker(1979)*.

SEXCAPADES

Alison Worth(pool babe)would likewise reappear as an
Octopussy girl in *Octopussy(1983)*.

§

Sensational chase scenes figured greatly in this superlative flick—too much so though. Stuntman Paolo Rigon was
tragically killed while filming the bobsled track portion of
the ski chase when his sled overturned, trapping him beneath, mortally injuring him.

Saturday night the 23rd of August 1980 I survived a
potentially deadly aspiring superspy's chase scene involving
ruthless assassins of my own!

"Stop, or I'll shoot you, mother fucker!"

That vulgar threat and command had been issued by a
scruffy and uncouth white youth standing next to a white
pickup truck—in the cab of which sat two beer–drinking
cohorts—at the edge of the spacious mall parking lot I was
passing by while biking northbound against traffic on the
southbound shoulder of the four–lane University Highway
road. In his hand the hoodlum was holding and pointing
straight at me a glistening hand*gun!*

Rather than stop I promptly sped up—pedaling hard toward the upcoming Interstate 10 overpass, leaving the hoodlum in the lurch!

Visibly vexed the snubbed hoodlum jumped in behind the
wheel and promptly peeled out in their screeching pickup to
give chase. I kept on pedaling hard northbound. Right off
though I observed the pursuing pickup, speeding likewise
northbound, pass by me on the opposite side of the highway. Ahead of me I watched the pickup U–turn at a gap in
the median strip at the upcoming interstate spur. Obviously
they undertook to overtake and head me off with the oncoming southbound traffic. But I kept my head—and my
wits about me!

Audaciously I crossed over the highway amidst breaks in the two lanes of oncoming southbound traffic to the opposite side, having to hurriedly uplift the bike and leap myself over the double median strip guardrails to make it safely and unscathed to the opposite shoulder of the road! In the meantime the *blundering* hoodlums were forced to pass by me again, speed all the way back to the mall parking lot exit from which they'd just emerged and U–turn again at the median–strip break in the highway to resume their hot pursuit! *Idiots!*

By then it was way too late for them to ever catch up to me. I kept on pedaling hard until I coasted calmly on my bike back across the highway's southbound lanes and into the parking lot of a well–lighted, well–populated, open–all–night, yellow logo *Waffle House* diner, where I promptly dialed *911* at a public pay phone to summon a promptly–responding county cop.

By that time the *blundering* hoodlums had to U–turn yet again at the interstate spur median–strip gap to cruise by the diner.

"C'mon, mother fuckers!" I yelled, waving them over.

"Mother fucker!" they yelled back, speeding off down the highway along with the swift–moving southbound traffic.

"Fuck you!" I yelled back last, flipping them the finger.

An aspiring superspy never seems to be packing his .25 Beretta automatic with skeleton grip precisely when he needs one!

Waffle House chain roadside restaurants—with at last count 1500 diners located in 25 states—remain something of a regional cultural icon throughout the southern United States; so it was rather ironic that I should take safe refuge there from hot pursuing hoodlums.

Purportedly the world's leading server of waffles, *USDA Choice* hamburgers, T–bone steaks, pork chops, patty melts, omelets, apple butter, cheese 'n eggs, grits, country ham, hashbrowns, raisin toast and traditional *Heinz 57* steak sauce, not to mention two percent of the eggs cracked in the nation's food service industry, where waitresses resort to diner lingo to call in orders for hashed brown potatoes—capped(with mushrooms), chunked(with diced ham), covered(with cheese), diced(with tomatoes), peppered(with jalapeño), scattered(spread over the grill), smothered(with onions), topped(with chili)and all the way(with all available toppings), it's a particularly sentimental safe house for me.

Opening first on Labor Day Weekend in 1955 at 2719 East College Avenue just outside Avondale Estates, Georgia that casual dine–in restaurant was along with Tom Forkner co–founded by *Joe* Rogers, *Sr*, who'd started out working as a short–order cook in 1947 in New Haven, Connecticut and later on as a regional manager in 1949 in Atlanta, Georgia for the now–defunct Memphis, Tennessee–based *Toddle House* restaurant chain, for which my own beloved father—*Joseph Sr*—likewise worked in the early 1960s in Hollywood and Jacksonville, Florida! So perhaps some paternal instinct drove me to seek asylum at *Waffle House!*

§

"That bank teller was *really* looking at you!" my cute and chubby black retail sales clerk from the mall bookstore, Bridget, confided protectively once I accompanied her to nearby *Barnett Bank* to make a deposit Wednesday morning the 3rd of September 1980. "I thought she was going to say something. But I was going to tell *her*: 'Not *my* Dicky, you don't! Get your *own* Dicky!"

§

Monday the 22nd of December before Christmas 1980 second–rate actress *Susan Walden* came traipsing into the mall bookstore where I worked, dispatching me to gift–wrap a couple of purchased books for her as presents. Second-rate, I say, solely because her sporadic career of supporting appearances in mostly television serials lasted roughly 15 years from 1977 to 1993 before fizzling out altogether. By that Christmas though she'd appeared in perhaps seven mediocre productions at best, so she acted conspicuously perturbed—expressing "hurt feelings" no less!—when I hadn't immediately recognized her prancing into the bookstore, her considerably aged face grotesquely rouged, as little *Miss Hollywood*(she'd already been a little "Florida Junior Miss" pageant contestant).

"Your face is so pink with make–up I didn't recognize you," I told her rather bluntly—diplomacy having never been my strong suit.

"It's just me," she proclaimed somewhat speciously.

She indulged in the excessively superficial niceties of asking how I was and whether I was ready for Christmas— "I'll never be," I joked—before I bid her a rather terse good-bye, delegating the closing of her transaction to a co–worker since Cindy was then coming into the store to greet me for my work–break, leaving Susan looking rather flustered.

Susan had been a drum majorette in my high school band and as a freshman had been my platonic girlfriend throughout my junior year until she inexplicably jilted me before subsequently transferring to local *Tate High School*—becoming, yes, a "Tater"—during my senior year when I took up with junior Regina. So she doubtless expected but was supremely shocked when I hadn't rolled out the red–carpet treatment for her upon making her grand entrance into the bookstore.

Sorry about that, Susan, but I've never been the fawning type!

§

"I think it shows the composite manifestation of your mentality," bellyached a black, turning pseudo–intellectual, who questioned my customer service response to his request for information at the mall bookstore Monday the 29th of December 1980.

"I think how you're acting now demonstrates yours," I retorted simply.

End of conversation!

§

So between doing back and forth both Cindy, who'd told me I was "so easy to be good to," and my Chinese girl-friend—not to mention my little love–nest coterie of recurring screwing–companions(reduced to Dalles and Jenny)—both familiar and strange—life in 1981 was in full, frenzied and frazzled swing! Cindy had abated some of the sexual stress by renting by mid–March a room off–campus in a house on Zelda Lane, where the amiable landlord named Buddy stipulated once–a–week "conjugal visits," which we typically engaged in either in Cindy's room or on their carpeted living room floor—though what with all the active coitus I'd be busy going at in the interim I scarcely caught up with Cindy again until the last day of May!

"You're easy to be good to," Cindy told me sweetly Thursday the 22nd of January 1981.

Jenny had subsequently moved as well to an off–campus duplex where I did her sporadically on her folding daybed in her living room into early 1982.

§

On April Fool's day at the nearby off–campus *Lil' General* convenience store I chatted up a buxom blond cashier–clerk named Ann(another nympho!)who treated me to a complimentary *Coke* and *Hershey* bar block.

By Thursday the 7th of May 1980 Ann would be visit-ing me at my private dormitory room on–campus follow-ing my theatrical performance in the historical city play for the so–called Galvez Celebration(3–10 May 1981), *I, Alone*, commemorating the Battle of Pensacola(March–8 May 1781), in which I was both acting as the play's principal antagonist(Admiral Don José Calbo)and playing entre'acte flugelhorn solos. She came bearing the gifts of a bottle of *Seagram VO* Canadian whiskey along with some chips, invit-ing me out to "party" the following Saturday, Indian-giving everything and unceremoniously leaving once my Chinese girlfriend came banging at my door late well past midnight!

After my third night of romping at my private dormitory room in mid–May with another fresh chick named Margaret, Ann called me to visit her off–campus at the *Lil' General* convenience store where she again treated me to a compli-mentary *Coke*, *Hershey* bar block and roast beef sandwich, gossiping about some rocker boyfriend and her ex–husband still pestering her to re–marry him.

Two nights after that, Friday the 15th of May 1981, fol-lowing a short stop at the *Moorings Apartments* on Old Spanish Trail Road to briefly visit a recently married girlfriend and have another drink of *Seagram VO* and cola, she drove the three of us to drink and dance at a club called *Machine Gun Kelly's* where she treated me to a couple of rum and colas. Out on the club's rearmost outdoor patio she tried goading me into smoking a joint, which I duly declined. Delivering her girlfriend home after the club closed she drove us back to my private dormitory room, I was promptly bonking her headlong in my bed, groping her bloated boobs with both hands when she abruptly hastened to get up and go before I could even get off! And just as abruptly after Ann left, I telephoned Cindy to come and babysit me all night, my head suddenly swirling with dizzying delirium until I finally passed out, sinking into mind–numbing oblivion. I wouldn't do dope so at some point, I suspected, Ann had slipped me a Mickey—though it wouldn't be until Saturday the 27th of June 1981 at the *Lil' General* store when Ann would treat me to another complimentary *Coke*, saying she'd swear "on a stack of Bibles" that she hadn't drugged my drink the night we'd partied!

Thus comforted *that*'d certainly made me feel better—especially by the beginning of July when she suddenly changed my complimentary à la carte menu to *Coke* and chips!

§

Following our cast rehearsal Thursday night the 30th of April 1981 the community play's leading lady, singer ***Debbie Mann***(playing the role of Felecia de Gálvez), asked me to escort her to her car, carrying along her reel–to–reel tape player and recorder. Once outside she brazenly and zealously French–kissed me, telling me that I should've been playing the production's lead protagonist and hero, Bernardo de Gálvez, rather than its antagonist and villain.
"*Dicky darling,*" Debbie wrote on my playbill, "*It was wonderful working with you. Hope to again, soon! 'Felecia'* ***Debbie Mann.***"

Thank you very much, Debbie! And my compliments to your *husband!*

Most significantly, Escambia High School's band director Wednesday the 6th of May 1981 offered me ten bucks an hour to teach trumpet to his novice student band members—some of whom performed the play's musical score!

Saturday the 23rd of May 1981, following a farm picnic cast party, a chick named Linda drove me home in her family's white van to my private dorm room on UWF campus.

"I want to stay out late and I'm determined to have fun!" she proclaimed suggestively.

At my place I kissed her profusely and promptly undid her blouse, uplifted her bra and led her to my bed where we necked feverishly, but she wouldn't fuck or even let me paw her pussy.

"No, no," she pleaded deliriously, "please don't."

On a second try I warmly massaged her back, kissing her neck, cheek and face, undid her blouse, uplifted her bra and we made out more until I pulled a sheet over us, peeled off my own clothes, nestling nude with her until she left, draping her in my own robe before she dressed and I saw her off.

§

Following my theatrical performance in the *Galvez* festival celebration play on that get lucky–and–score Wednesday the 8th of May 1980, Margaret, the cute, busty and freckled young blond sister of one of my fellow histrionic cast members, accompanied me to a downtown ad agency's night-time cocktail party in a renovated Victorian house on Baylen Street to which our show's cast had been duly invited. After so much drunken revelry and merry–making we soon found ourselves sitting together outside, warmly embraced on the front porch swing seethingly "sucking face" as one passing observer bluntly put it.

Margaret invited me to visit more privately at her nearby house at 118 West Gadsden Street for which we directly headed together on foot. On our way I abruptly and impulsively took Margaret by her hand, leading the way into the darkened and secluded section of an expansive backyard to another huge house, grabbing her ample rump tightly with both hands and plunking her down behind some dense shrubbery at the foot of a hefty *ole* oak tree—but not to tie any yellow ribbons!—where I impetuously yanked up her bra and top, promptly exposing her plump and supple breasts to both the moonlight and my grasp, uplifted her short skirt, stripped off her scanty panties—my rock–hard rod bursting out of my pants at the zipper—then forcefully and repeatedly plunged and pumped her spurting wet pussy to her stifled outcries until we both finally went limp and breathless with the rippling, surging explosion of all my cream!

After stopping by her house only briefly later on, Margaret drove us both to my private dormitory room on–campus where I fucked her forcefully not once but *twice* more before she made a discreet exit out of the south wing of the building while my Chinese girlfriend would clamor to enter the west wing!

Margaret was white–hot stuff; the next time I got into her pants at her house three nights later on Sunday the 11th the peeled legs of her jeans never got past her pale ankles! She was back friskily fucking me on Wednesday the 13th at my private dormitory room two nights after that. Six nights after that on Tuesday the 19th we were getting it on together in her roomy car parked at a darkened curb in my old *East Hill* neighborhood—then back at the dormitory five nights after that(between nights with Jenny before and after Margaret)on Sunday the 24th! Five nights after that on Friday the 29th we parked her car at the off–campus *Fountains Ltd.* Apartments on University Parkway so we could go screw in the woods where I'd go with my mall groupie, Jackie, near the *Nativity of Our Lord Catholic Church* at 9945 Hillview Drive.

§

Wednesday night the 3rd of June 1980, speaking of getting down and dirty on the solid ground, I was invited to attend a birthday party at the well–traversed downtown *Sheraton Inn*, where I rather drunkenly hooked up with an older lady visiting from Tuscumbia, Alabama named Myra, the dishy elder of a mother–and–daughter duo.

"I bet you're fantastic," she demurred modestly when we diverted briefly to the beach, where I laid her down to *get* laid, "but this isn't private."

So I followed the duo driving their sky–blue *Bobcat* off North Davis Highway, conveniently enough near the university environs, to indeed the more remote and secluded dirt–road located daughter's house—behind which I again laid down comely Myra, peeling off her jeans and panties and pumping her good right there on the darkened ground.

"It was good!" Myra kept on repeating as I walked her to the house's doorstep before seeing myself off with a sweet and soft kiss.

Three nights after that on Saturday the 6th I was back getting it on with Margaret in her car parked on a secluded dirt–road space behind the University Mall–proximate *Holiday Inn Express* on Plantation Road—replaced today by *Residence* and *Red Roof Inns* at 7230–7340 Plantation Road!

At the time then dirt roads were coming in pretty damn handy!

Friday night the 26th of June 1980 Margaret drove us off Pace Boulevard to an abandoned nursery overgrown with weeds and brushwood called the "ghost town" where she parked her car where we could screw until we were both bathed in sweat!

On the eve of July 4th 1980 we were heatedly humping in her room back at her house. Seven nights later we were getting more over–heated auto–action parked on a deserted road close to campus. Friday the 24th of July 1980 we got on some blood–hot ass together parked in Margaret's steamed–up car amidst all the other numerous parked cars belonging to residents at the university–proximate *Azalea Trace Retirement Community* likewise on Hillview Drive, where on our way out we got busted still drenched in sweat by a prowling county deputy sheriff who was only mildly amused when I told him we'd been...*sightseeing!*

Well, I *had* been sightseeing in the lamplight—Margaret's ample, supple and swelling breasts, so wet to the skin, so fervid to the warm squeeze of my feverishly caressing and groping hot hands.

Monday the 17th of August 1980 Margaret dropped by to greet me at the mall bookstore toward the end of my night workshift, and what with only one other co–worker on duty cashiering up at the storefront, I secreted Margaret into the rear stockroom, hoisted her up atop the wooden worktable, spread her thickset thighs in front of me, inserting myself between her knees attempting to penetrate her with my prong though the angle of contact was rather high and her shrunken shorts extremely constricting.

So after work I pulled my already once previously successful ploy of taking Margaret along with me during that particular term break to the on–campus marital dormitories, where I admitted us with my kept key to the crazed Cuban–American witch's old apartment for another of our steamy–hot and sweaty sessions on the old marital bed!

"I'll play around with you anytime," she sweetly complimented me. "You're really good to be with!"

"If only the ex–wife could see me now," I mused aloud.

"She'd probably want to kill you."

"She wouldn't care," I said with a more sober disposition. "But we hadn't better press our luck here. I don't believe we'd pass for the housing staff!"

Margaret laughed aloud as she dressed and spruced herself up to leave.

We met up to get it on again Friday the 28th of August 1980 for another woodsy footpath tryst, breaking in Saturday the 5th of September 1980 back at my private dormitory room.

By mid–August 1981 the university conferred on me its third equally worthless bachelor of arts(BA)degree in international studies, so–called.

DICKY GALORE

§

Biking back to the university on the night of September 11th, 1981(20 years to the day *before* that terrifying 9/11 in 2001)I stopped by the *Lil' General* convenience store and happened upon a verbal altercation–in progress between a grumpy drunken older man and a corpulent but comely young blond chick whose name I presently came to find out was Teresa and who drove me back to campus for a hot tryst in the woods!

It was one of those senseless, contentious face–offs between young and old:

"What are you lookin' at?" she said.

"I'm lookin' at you!" he said.

"You can't look at me!" she said.

"It's a free country," he said, "I'll look at whoever I want!"

Et Cet'era, et cet'era, et cet'era!!!

Since she was already frisky and well worked up, it was pretty easy to entice Teresa to drive me—and my bike—back to campus where she directly let me lead her straight down the dark garden path and into those grassy and mossy woods! Before long she was flat on her back, her pants peeled, her legs spread wide open, her plump pink breasts bursting and bouncing in the moonlight, her squealing voice crying out aloud while I pumped her repeatedly with my long hard prong, pressing both of my palms upward against the warm undersides of her thickset thighs to uplift her juicy, peachy wet pussy to swallow me whole even more!

"You're so good!" she so sweetly complimented me. "Such a fantastic lover!"

Teresa promptly stopped by the mall bookstore during my workshift to greet me the very next evening so she must've meant it!

§

SEXCAPADES

By Sunday the 11th of October 1980 I'd already moved across town close to the local junior college to shack up with my Chinese girlfriend in an efficiency apartment, so–called, at the *Lamplighter Apartments* at 711 Underwood Avenue. But I was still antsy to assert my aspiring superspy manly virility.

So late Wednesday night the 28th of October 1980 I hit up on Langley Avenue at the nearby *Tom Thumb Food Store* its buxom brunet lady manager named Rosemarie, who I presently invited out after closing at eleven o'clock to help me drink a bottle of rotgut wine I just bought from her there.

Surprisingly Rosemarie was exceptionally obliging and all ready to go! So much so that she readily volunteered to drive us in her *Dodge* pickup truck to a secluded spot at the foot of Langley Avenue intersecting Scenic Highway over-looking placid *Escambia Bay* from the abrupt, lofty bluffs. There in the rather cramped quarters of her cab I hastily got into Rosemarie's pants between her fleshy thickset thighs and banged her sloppy wet pussy good right up against the cab's passenger door—after which she drove me back home in fine fettle!

Throughout the fall term at the junior college from August through December 1981 I attended and successfully completed with a #1 award in physical training its police recruit academy #37, so–called, earning its law enforcement certificate sanctioned by Florida's *Commission on Criminal Justice Standards and Training*.

§

Now I know what you're thinking: that was a mighty *LOT* of screwing around in 1981! Well, yes it was—and to coin a more contemporary hood phrase—it was a whole hec-ka–hella *LOT* of fun too! But consider the times in which it all went down.

Throughout the footloose and fancy–freewheeling 1970s—treading right on the hot heels of the swinging 1960s—lots of horny chicks were hot to trot and ever ready to get down and profusely *rock!* I for one was there all ready to accommodate as many of them as I could! And best of all they were mostly all *on the pill* so there was none of this ever so silly politically correct *stuff and nonsense* as there still stupidly persists today about extremely *UN*–natural "safe sex," so–called, condoms, and dudes "sharing the responsibility" for exclusively maternal birth control!

Our Bodies, Ourselves was the classic 1970s profoundly feminist *Boston Women's Health Book Collective* women's health manifesto of the time and succinctly summarized what at least ought to be women's ***SOLE AND EXCLUSIVE RESPONSIBILITY FOR THEIR OWN PREVENTIVE BIRTH CONTROL IDENTICALLY EQUAL TO THEIR SOLE AND EXCLUSIVE RESPONSIBILITY FOR THEIR OWN POST–PREGNANCY REPRODUCTIVE RIGHTS***, so–called. There simply exists no *true* "shared responsibility" for what is truly every individual woman's *sole* and *exclusive* responsibility: the condition of *HER* body, *HER*–self!

Today's *HYPOCRITICALLY*–correct chicks would palm off onto their copulating "partners" that responsibility by refusing to assume it *fully*—*THEIR* bodies, *THEIR*–selves!! Sorry, ladies, but you can't have it both ways: you can't claim sole and exclusive reproductive "rights" to aborting babies without equally and fully claiming sole and exclusive ***RESPONSIBILITIES*** for *controlling births* of babies!

So don't try so lamely to fob off onto your dudes those responsibilities which you must *solely* and *exclusively* assume—for *YOUR* bodies, *YOUR*–selves! And if you really crave to fuck but really crave likewise to prevent getting pregnant, then either get on some truly effective birth control or else keep your hot slutty thighs *shut* and outright ***REFUSE*** that ejaculating dick's pussy–of–entry! After all, unless you're criminally raped, no sperm–spewing dick shoots off in *YOUR* body's pussy without *YOUR*–self's own free and willing *CONSENT—for which in the end there is ultimately no "partnering" or "sharing!"*

Taking exclusive and full RESPONSIBILITY of YOUR body YOUR–self is REAL womanly "empowerment!"

As for resorting to condoms, that's not just *non*sense, it's *un*natural *NON*–sex and for the moment we won't even go there. Suffice it to say, I've never, *ever* once resorted to the artificial artifice of condoms and never *ever* shall! Suffice it to say as well, horny chicks throughout the 1970s were truly hot to trot—and they not only did fucking *good*, they did fucking *RIGHT!* Trust me, then, I ought to know—I was there doing it good and right...right along *with* them with their full and unfettered consent and participation!

It wasn't until 5 June 1981 that the Centers for Disease Control and Prevention reported that five *homosexual* men in Los Angeles, California contracted a rare form of pneumonia afflicting only patients suffering weakened immune systems: the first recognized cases of the **AIDS**(Acquired Immune Deficiency Syndrome)resulting from the **HIV**(human immunodeficiency virus)! That subsequent terroristic sexual *SCARE*—and the extremely *EXAGGERATED* and *over*blown threat to healthy and natural *hetero*sexual sex—put of course the unduly discouraging "chilling effect" damper on good old–fashioned fucking by means of sexual *PARANOIA*–provoking *PROPAGANDA* which tragically and tenaciously persists to this present day!

But as you'll see, while he boldly went in 1982 where no dick had ever gone before, **Dicky Galore** kept right on fucking *UN*–dissuaded and *UN*–deterred as decades later he still does even *today: condom–and–disease–free!*

Live long and prosper—fuck free and fuck a LOT!

§

Following our simple civil marriage in August 1981 I relocated together with my Chinese girlfriend by the end of May 1982 to the state capital of Tallahassee, Florida—some 200 miles east in the central state panhandle—where she would continue her studies at *Florida State University(FSU)*. Before we pulled up stakes in Pensacola, Florida though I had one final affair—albeit a somewhat embarrassing one.

Monday the 22nd of February 1982 at *Cordova Mall* at 5100 North 9th Avenue I happened upon a casual acquaintance of mine from the nearby junior college, a cute and tender brunet named Judy. Together we sauntered about the shops, she treated me to a *Coke* at the *Montgomery Ward* chain department store, and the next day the 23rd we strolled about the college campus, going along between the library and the golf putting green near the running track with her much comelier sister, Mary, becoming better acquainted.

Thursday the 25th of February 1982 I met up again with Judy, sporting her dark blue white—striped sweat suit, and we went jogging together along the trails amidst the piny woods bordering the college campus. Naturally we paused at the foot of some pine tree to take a breather doing some breathless necking and petting before calling it an afternoon, drinking *Coke* back at nearby *Cordova Mall*'s *Montgomery Ward* chain department store.

Saturday the 20th of March 1982 I ran into Judy and her sister, Mary, at the *Westwood Mall*; they invited me to visit their family(Grimes–Williams)at their house in the nearby *Montclair* neighborhood at 1012 Fairmont Drive, where I pressed their step–father's 85–pound barbell in their den 24 times; he spotted me for a 25th lift. *Montclair* was another working–class neighborhood adjoining my childhood neighborhood of *Mayfair*.

Wednesday the 7th of April 1982 I got invited again to

their home for a hearty supper of spaghetti, pot roast, mashed potatoes and string beans.

Easter Sunday the 11th of April 1982 I rode over to their house to give Judy the token gift of a small yellow stuffed Easter chick.

Before long though it became inscrutably clear that the strongest and most enticing attraction was drawing me more toward not Judy but rather her lovely, dark–haired, large–eyed, luscious–lipped sister, Mary, who was but a tender teen of 18!

Monday the 12th of April 1982 Mary and I found ourselves alone and on our own together at their house, where we were warmly embraced and making out, sitting astride her step–father's flat weight–training bench in the sunken den of their house. Partly stripped—her scanty panties were shed, my prong was out, long, rigid and throbbing to penetrate her—I laid Mary gently down lengthwise along the bench. One of my hands softly groped one of her plump and supple breasts while the crook of my other arm, curled behind one of her bent knees, uplifted one of her legs, spreading her thickset thighs wide open to take me in.

No sooner had my hardened head and shaft plunged deep into her gushing wet honeypot did Mary, making a wry face, cry out with a panicky gasp and abruptly struggle to wriggle free from impalement. Looking powerfully apprehensive Mary abruptly got up to guide us together into her bedroom where she doffed the rest of her garments, offering to model for me her newest string bikini to tempt and tantalize me further! Before long then I was on her bed lying atop her, groping her ample bosom and piercing her sopping pussy right through her writhing bikini bottom!

At one jump though Mary suddenly bounded from her bed, blocking her bedroom door to bar entry to her youngest sister, Connie, who'd returned home unexpectedly to surprise—and *bust*—us!

DICKY GALORE

I made a discreet and hasty exit, and I even paid them another jovial visit at their house Thursday the 15th of April 1982, for yet another dinner date, before their entire family of five—mother, step–father and three daughters—stopped by en masse to pay me a painfully solemn visit at the new *Cordova Mall Waldenbooks* store where I'd recently been recruited to work part–time while tutoring adult basic education students at the nearby junior college. Connie had blabbed and ratted Mary and me out!

Suffice it to say, that Saturday the 17th of April 1982 I was quietly and seriously cautioned under no uncertain terms never to set foot on their doorstep ever again.

Yes, I was politely but firmly dressed down by their step–father, Albert Williams. No, I wasn't cursed or menaced, nor would I've suffered myself to be. But it was a mightily embarrassing moment and I was duly and most humbly repentant.

§

In 1982, a rather rueful year for an aspiring superspy, Austrian actor of German–French ancestry, Curt Jergens, who played the villainous Karl Stromberg, the sociopathic industrialist seeking to transform the planet into an ocean paradise in the *Spy Who Loved Me(1977)*, tragically died June 18th after suffering a heart attack.

SIX:
OCTOWUSSY

"Nothing you have ever expressed to me has ever sounded silly even your infatuation with **James Bond**.*"—*

Regina, 5 September 1973

Octopussy(1983), starring once more Sir Roger Moore as not–so–secret British agent, James Bond 007, was naturally pitted against Sir Sean Connery's reluctant return to the role in the "unofficial" *Never Say Never Again(1983)*, released of course in the very same year in what was dubbed at the time as the so–called "Battle of the Bonds." Well, with all due respect to Sir Sean Connery's superlative creation of the role, Sir Roger Moore's Bond handily won that particular battle— hands down! As has been duly documented he won single– handedly at the box office as well.

For me it wasn't so much which actor was the better Bond—as both future knights of the realm had by then nearly equally established themselves in the role even though in vastly different respects—as it was which was, forgive the pun, the *Moore FUN* and enjoyable film!

Despite some excruciatingly silly sequences—not the least of which included Bond decked out in a clown costume and *Octopussy's* bevy of bikini–clad "cult" chick acrobats overpowering a contingent of heavily armed palace guards— in one of those outrageously gratuitous displays of *wistful* feminist thinking!, much akin to those two extremely runty "martial artist" schoolgirls in that ridiculous dojo escape scene from the *Man with the Golden Gun(1974)*—in terms of sheer charm, humor and entertainment Moore's Bond smoothly surpassed Connery's Bond in almost every respect. So sorry about that, Sir Sean!

Then there was the deservedly hit–making title theme song, *"All Time High,"* sung so sensitively by Rita Coolidge in top velvety voice. And then there was the incredibly stun- ning Miss Sweden(1970)/Miss Universe semi–finalist/Miss Scandinavia–turned–actress, Kristina Wayborn, playing the devastating villainess, Magda.

Reportedly Austrian actress Sybil Danning was the first choice publicly announced to be cast as *Octopussy*. In retrospect Sybil's far more powerful(and carnal)presence would've proved to be eminently superior to the comparatively insipid personality of Maud Adams while yet preserving the exceptionally exotic flavor of the cast.

Douglas Wilmer(Jim Fanning)'s a celebrated veteran of both classical fantasy and horror films, appearing amongst them most impressively in *Jason and the Argonauts(1963)*as Pelias, *The Brides of Fu Manchu (1966)*and *The Vengeance of Fu Manchu* (1967)as Nayland Smith, *The Vampire Lovers(1970)* as Baron Joachim von Hartog, *The Golden Voyage of Sinbad (1974)*as the Vizier, as well as in two Pink Panther films, *A Shot In The Dark(1964)*as Henri LaFarge and *Revenge of the Pink Panther(1978)*as the Police Commissioner.

Philip Voss(the auctioneer)played Ernst in *Hammer Horror's Frankenstein and the Monster from Hell(1974)*.

Peter Porteous(Lenkin)would return in *The Living Daylights(1987)*as the gasworks supervisor.

Stuart Saunders(Major Clive)appeared in two notable horror flicks, *The Trollenberg Terror(1958)*as Dewherst and *Horrors of the Black Museum(1959)*as the Strength-Test Barker as well as in two flicks starring a striking 31–year–old pre–James Bond Sean Connery in *Frightened City(1961)*as Publican and *On The Fiddle(1961)*as Sarge.

Patrick Barr(British Ambassador)likewise played along with Sir Sean in *The Longest Day(1962)*, uncredited as Group Captain JN Stagg, as well as *Hammer Horror's The Satanic Rites of Dracula(1974)*as Lord Carradine and two less noteworthy horrors, *The Flesh and Blood Show(1972)*as Major Bell/ Sir Arnold Gates and *The House of Whipcord(1974)*as Justice Bailey.

Gertan Klauber(Bubi)played the Tavernkeeper in the noteworthy Vincent Price horror flick, *Cry of the Banshee(1970)*.

Richard Graydon(Francisco the Fearless)also appeared fearlessly in *You Only Live Twice(1967)*as the Russian

SEXCAPADES

Spacecraft Astronaut and *On Her Majesty's Secret Service(1969)* as Draco's driver.

Ishaq Bux(Fakir)had already appeared notably as Fakir in *Amicus'* horror anthology, *The Vault of Horror(1973)*.

Eugene Lipinski(Head VOPO, uncredited)played Cane, the Elevator Suicide, in Sean Connery's *Outland(1981)*.

Stunning Hammer Horror babe of *Vampire Lovers(1970)* as Marcilla/Carmilla/Mircalla Karnstein and *Countess Dracula(1971)*as Countess Elisabeth Nodosheen fame, Ingrid Pitt, performed *Octopussy's* uncredited Galley Mistress voice! Ingrid's likewise notably remembered for her performances in *Amicus' The House That Dripped Blood(1971)*as Carla Lynde and *The Omegans(1968)*as Linda.

Never Say Never Again(1983), by contrast, is a remissfully comatose remake of *Thunderball(1965)*riddled with ludicrous and lacklustrous *mis*–casting: a nonsensical "M," a bland "Blofeld"—and despite all his *over*–hyped but *non*–existent charm and charisma—an incredibly insipid "Largo" played to an almost flamingly effeminate extent by Klaus "Maria" Brandauer, who thank **GOD** was never cast as Connery's Marko Ramius in the *Hunt for the Red October(1990)*! Equally banal was Kim Basinger as "Domino"—as was the irritatingly politically correct casting of a conspicuously complacent footballer–actor Bernie Casey as a black CIA chum, "Felix Leiter!" Added to all that the adolescent antics of pre–"Mr Bean," Rowan Atkinson, as inept "Nigel Small–Fawcett"—who might've just as well been renamed Nigel Dripping Tap!—and this flick's calamitous *mis*–casting was altogether complete!

From that completely preposterous and pointless Arab slave–market escape sequence on it was a headlong downward slide to that flick's deadly *dull* denouement!

Mind you, the movie did have its precious few rare moments: Barbara Carrera as strikingly flamboyant "Fatima Blush" easily stole the villainess show just as her sumptuous co–support stars Prunella Gee("Patricia")and Valerie Leon(Bahamas Babe)stole the sexually erotic scenery! Why, even Alec McCowen(of "Mr. Palfrey of Westminster" fame) came through brilliantly as "Algernon" of "Q" branch!

Apart from Sir Sean Connery's consistently dashing depiction of Bond, though, his was a rather *weak sister* compared to Sir Roger Moore's consistently courtly portrayal in 1983!

§

TRICKY DICK

In 1950 Richard M Nixon was elected to the United States Senate, defeating Congresswoman Helen Gahagen Douglas, accusing her of harboring communist sympathies and dubbing her the "Pink Lady," jesting that she was "pink right down to her underwear." Gahagen, in turn, christened Nixon with one of the most enduring nicknames in politics: *Tricky Dick!!*

Now I know what ya'll are really wondering: how big— or small—is it and does size really matter? Well, I'm most inclined to agree with one celebrated prostitute who essentially said: it matters to those to whom it matters!

What I also know matters is indeed *how* you use it—how you move it, how you position it, what you do with it, when, where, and with what rapidity or delay. And there's no pre-set formula for that except, as with most everything else, patient practice and experience.

Another thing I know for sure is that it's almost always a superior practice to intuitively and spontaneously *feel* and *do* sex in a free, unforced and unstrained manner rather than mechanically and robotically talk, direct or otherwise laboriously *exercise* sex with lots of excessively self–conscious(and unnatural)"communication," so in fashion amongst today's politically correct but sexually neurotic automatons. Corresponding *body* language is, after all, the supreme method of sexual communication. Just **DO** it, shut the fuck up and fuck!

From personal experience—and after *scads* of screwing—all I can safely say is: the dick truly is a remarkably *tricky* thing and no dick functions or performs in the exact same way—to the exact same *extent*, as it were—each and every time *all* the time. And any cocky boasting to the contrary is—as are the high–flown sexploits of super secret agent James Bond 007—sheer fabulous and fanciful **FANTASY!**

A really robust, vigorous and virile dick is primarily a matter of freely running blood flow which hangs in turn on a healthy state of emotional, mental, physical and spiritual fitness. So no dick is helping his case any by doing drugs, smoking, drinking to excess, neglecting healthful and wholesome nutrition, and failing to ever exercise and work out.

Under certain awkward or uncomfortable circumstances—or even colder extremes of temperature—mine's petered out, so to speak, and shrunk up to next to nothing. Properly provoked and stimulated, on the other hand, it's duly swollen and shot up to mightily throbbing lengths. Equally essential to the hottest and most vital sex then is that sheer but inexplicable chemistry experienced with that special inspirational partner perceived to be the most appetizing, provocative and tantalizing. Impassioned love and lust combined inflames the blood to its feverishly highest boiling points!

So never permit an impatient, inconsiderate or otherwise unsympathetic pussy to ever blame your dick unduly for going limp from suffering that temporary bout of sexual dysfunction. More often than not a suddenly dysfunctional dick is afflicted with either outright fatigue—or else is confronted with a profoundly *UN*–appealing and *UN*–inspirational partner.

So not to worry—there's no secret esoteric mystery to what ought to be so blatantly obvious: enjoying the hottest and most satisfying sex swings in the end on finding—and fucking—the most *mutually* desir*ous* as well as the most desir*able* partner!

§

Speaking of aesthetic tastes and sensibilities, I've doubtless scored and screwed more and more varied chicks of every conceivable stripe, coloration and description than fictional creator Ian Fleming's superspy could've ever envisioned. Talk about "diversity!" So my eminently immature high school sweetheart, Regina—who after cavorting together for several years knew me so little after all—was wholly wrong: I was never "infatuated" so much with James Bond as such as with the consummately masculine, criminally handsome and inimitably talented Scottish cinema star who single–handedly embodied and personified him so perfectly: the impeccable and incomparable ***SEAN CONNERY!***

Every man wants to *be* him and every man wants to *do* it *like* him!

Compared to my high school sweetheart, Regina, or for that matter my Cuban–American witch of a wife, Elizabeth, who idolized respectively the likes of either actors Kurt Russell or John Travolta, I feel quite confident in retrospect that my aesthetic taste in cinematic celebrity has proved to be their conspicuous superior.

So far Sir Sean Connery's been duly honored for his cinematic acting in more recent years with Academy(1987), BAFTA(1986)and Golden Globe(1988)awards, including the latter's Cecil B DeMille award(1996)as well as the Kennedy Center Honors(1999)for lifetime contributions to arts and culture, the European Film Award(2005)for lifetime achievement and the American Film Institute(AFI)'s

Lifetime Achievement Award(2006), amongst many others too numerous to mention.

Lest we forget, Queen Elizabeth II awarded him his Knighthood in July 2000!

Now I'm no pretentious *retro*–admirer of Sir Sean Connery, devoutly patronizing and supporting his films most *consistently* throughout my youth—throughout even the tacky 1970s when he was short–sightedly second–guessed by some misinformed circles to be some "box–office poison" has–been simply because he'd balked and passed up playing James Bond any further—even to the present day!

Every manly man's signs of course will have different meaning and differing degrees(and intensities)of importance to attach to such signs. So I'll close this chapter simply with my amicable admonition to manly men everywhere: remember always to ***read the signs!***

DICKY GALORE WILL BE BACK!
AND WILL RETURN IN:
SEXCAPADES BY THE DECADES:
THE THIRTIES

For the most part of both 1982 and 1983 I'd given Dicky Galore a well–deserved rest, settled down(albeit briefly)and focused instead—in the place of pumping Pussy Galore— on writing back–to–back two complimentary political tracts treating the twin subjects of war and peace. Only...*And War For All: The Pledge of Subjection(1983/2005)*ever made it to print.

By that time I'd been in definite danger of becoming—as Canadian actor Joseph Wiseman's "Dr No" would've put it— *"just a stupid policeman...whose luck has run out!"*—when all I've ever really aspired to be was just another stupid writer! But in October 1983 that writer's ideal dream computer pro- gram—*Microsoft Word*—had just been first released. Only time shall tell then whether I've ever actually succeeded at fulfilling that scrupulous and suspect aspiration.

In this volume I've deliberately skirted past steady long– term romantic relationships, preferring to recount those for another separate writing project altogether. Likewise I've purposely opted to postpone rendering a more explanatory account of Dicky Galore's previous juvenile and avant–garde exploits for yet another descriptive *prequel*. In the meantime, writing resumes on two graphic sexcapades *sequels* recount- ing anecdotally this aspiring superspy's *sex*ploits during the ensuing decades throughout both his thirties and forties.

Look out then for Dicky Galore's most forthcoming ti- tle—***Sexcapades by the Decades: The Thirties***—coming soon to an online internet retail bookseller near you! Those prom- ise to be the most shamelessly salacious and promiscuous of all!